THE
Healthy Pet
MANUAL

"I have given care to domestic animals for over 25 years and sadly, more than half of them have died with cancer. With *The Healthy Pet Manual* beside me, I feel more confident as I continue this work. I will now be better able to hopefully prevent cancer before it appears and also ease the way for those animals who already have cancer, coming into my family for quality end-of-life support. In this extraordinary volume, author Deborah Straw offers us one of the finest and most essential tools for providing optimum care to the animals we hold dear. I can't thank her enough for that."

RITA M. REYNOLDS,
AUTHOR OF *BLESSING THE BRIDGE:*
WHAT ANIMALS TEACH US ABOUT DEATH, DYING, AND BEYOND

"*The Healthy Pet Manual* is a must-read for those who consider their companion animals family members. This book considers all facets of our pets' health, including their emotional needs, and thus is a refreshing approach to keeping our four-legged kids healthy. If everyone showed the respect and consideration for animals that Deborah Straw demonstrates, we would not only have healthier animals, we would live in a world free of unwanted and abused animals. Two paws up!"

RANDY GRIM, AUTHOR OF *MIRACLE DOG,*
SUBJECT OF THE BOOK *THE MAN WHO TALKS TO DOGS,*
AND FOUNDER OF STRAY RESCUE OF ST. LOUIS.

"I have long encouraged pet owners to learn as much as they can about behavior so humans and pets can better communicate and live in harmony. The same emphasis should be on the health of your pets, including prevention and treatment. Deborah's *Healthy Pet Manual* deals openly with the changing world of animal healthcare including the causes of disease, amazing advances in care and treatment, and costs. Her insight is valuable for maintaining a healthy pet and provides a lot of transferable insight into human health."

MATTHEW "UNCLE MATTY" MARGOLIS,
WORLD-RENOWNED DOG TRAINER
AND HOST OF THE PBS SERIES *WOOF! IT'S A DOG'S LIFE*

THE
Healthy Pet
MANUAL

A Guide to the Prevention and
Treatment of Cancer

DEBORAH STRAW

Healing Arts Press
Rochester, Vermont

Healing Arts Press
One Park Street
Rochester, Vermont 05767
www.InnerTraditions.com

Healing Arts Press is a division of Inner Traditions International

Note to the reader: This book is intended as an informational guide. The remedies, approaches, and techniques described herein are meant to supplement, and not to be a substitute for, professional veterinary care or treatment. They should not be used to treat a serious ailment without prior consultation with a state-licensed veterinarian.

The Library of Congress has cataloged a previous edition of this title as follows:

Straw, Deborah.
    Why is cancer killing our pets?: how you can protect and treat your animal companion
      / Deborah Straw.
    p. cm.
    Includes bibliographical references and index.
    ISBN 0-89281-926-X
      1. Dogs—Diseases. 2. Cats—Diseases. 3. Pets—Diseases. 4. Cancer in animals.
    5. Holistic veterinary medicine. I. Title.

SF992.C35 S77 2005
636.7'0896994—dc21

                                                     00-059786

ISBN of current title *The Healthy Pet Manual:* ISBN 1-59477-057-3

Printed and bound in Canada by Transcontinental Printing

10   9   8   7   6   5   4   3   2   1

Text design and layout by Virginia L. Scott Bowman
This book was typeset in Sabon with Bauer Bodoni, Gill Sans, and Frutiger as the display typefaces

Dedicated to Puck, Bauhaus, Annie, and Misty

Contents

Foreword

When my sister-in-law was diagnosed with breast cancer three years ago, my wife's second trip was to the childhood home where she grew up, to spend time with her sibling. Her first trip was to the bookstore, where she bought several volumes with titles such as *What To Do When A Loved One Has Cancer*. There were dozens to choose from, designed to acquaint cancer patients and their families with the etiology of the disease, current treatments (with the risk of side effects), along with prognosis and survival rates. Many books also address the emotional and psychological aspects of facing serious illness: handling stress, communicating with friends and relatives, coping with depression, and maintaining hope. For many people, such books are a godsend, helping them through the initial period of shock and bewilderment as they gradually gain their bearings.

But what are your resources when the "loved one" you care for is a dog or cat or another animal companion? Our culture has tended to minimize the importance of the human-animal bond and to discount the stakes when a beloved pet becomes ill. The attitude that "it's only an animal" is still all too common. There are few books in the "pet" section that offer the same kind of information and support that are readily available in the "people" section of the bookstore. The volume you are now holding, Deborah Straw's *The Healthy Pet Manual* is one of the first and most comprehensive to address this important need.

A book such as this can be valuable in many ways. Foremost, it can help you ask more intelligent questions and become a better advocate for your pet. You'll be empowered to take charge of your animal's well-being and become a more responsible consumer of veterinary and pet care services. Read in time, a book like this might even save a life.

When my office manager was told her cat needed an ultrasound, for instance, her initial reaction was a feeling of helplessness and dependency. There was only one specialist in our area who provided this particular procedure for animals. She wasn't always sure she understood or agreed with all the treatment recommended, but where else could she turn? She was at the mercy of the system. No book can offer a substitute for the training and experience of a trusted vet. But a work like this one can enable you to make more informed decisions and better understand your options.

Deborah Straw encourages readers to ask a whole range of questions they may not have considered previously. What vaccines are necessary to protect your pet, and what risks are involved in most common vaccinations? How safe are commercial or premium brand pet foods? What are the pros and cons of purchasing insurance for your animal? The glossary and appendices alone would make this book a worthwhile addition to the pet lover's bookshelf. But the wealth of data and documentation within its pages make it an essential reference.

The Healthy Pet Manual covers both conventional and more holistic approaches to coping with cancer, which is a real strength, recognizing that people spend almost as much money today on alternative therapies as they do on conventional medical care. The two paradigms are not necessarily incompatible. One woman in my church, for instance, decided to follow her doctor's recommendation and go with radiation treatments after a lumpectomy, but complemented her reliance on high-tech medicine with visits to an acupuncturist (with the blessing of her physician), which she felt helped keep her energy level higher than it might have been. Most people, I think, want to consider all the possibilities when facing a potentially life-threatening situation, and this holds true whether we are concerned with people or pets. *The Healthy Pet Manual* offers a judicious and balanced exploration of everything from surgery to herbal remedies, with as much emphasis on prevention as on cure.

A book like this may also help you feel less frightened and alone.

Until we find that it has reached into our own homes, many of us believe that cancer is a disease that primarily afflicts "other people" (and other people's pets). Of course, the statistics prove otherwise. Cancer is the number one killer of dogs and cats. But when we find that cancer has invaded our own lives and the lives of those we love, our initial response can be denial and disbelief, followed by feelings of discouragement and isolation. Perhaps nothing quite like this has happened to us before. Friends and even other family members may have trouble relating to the experience.

How comforting it can be at such moments to find the voice of someone who truly sympathizes. The fact that the author has lost several of her own animal companions to cancer and related ailments makes her an especially sensitive guide to others in need, dispensing not only practical advice but also personal understanding. Studies have shown again and again that patients who are struggling with cancer have better odds of beating the disease when they have a strong network of support—people they can trust, who know what they're going through. And surely those who accompany their animals through illness can benefit from the company of an individual like Deborah Straw, whose caring and genuineness are evident in everything she writes.

I am pleased to count Deborah among my small circle of friends. She is a person who not only loves animals but has the soul of a poet, enabling her to speak eloquently on behalf of all the creatures who add such grace, beauty, and felicity to our human existence.

Yet this cannot have been an easy book for her to write. As a clergyman, I realize there is an inward cost to those who make it their business to address the realities of death, disease, and discomfort. But I also know that such work can be tremendously satisfying and rewarding, however difficult it may be. *The Healthy Pet Manual* is well worth the long hours and meticulous research that went into writing it and will certainly help the thousands of people who read it and find comfort and clarity within its covers.

Thank you, Deborah, for this timely contribution to the literature of healing.

GARY KOWALSKI
AUTHOR OF *THE SOULS OF ANIMALS*

Acknowledgments

I wish to thank the many people who helped me with this complex, important, and often heart-wrenching book. First, I want to thank my husband, Bruce Conklin, who read each draft of my manuscript and put up with my moods during the final weeks of the book's completion and its revision. He also fixed many computer snafus and helped with the tricky endnoting process. Without his encouragement and support, I could not have taken on this task. Thanks also go to my parents, Donald and Phyllis Straw, without whom I would not have developed such a strong love for and interest in all animals. Alice Wright, my beloved sister-in-law who died of cancer in summer 2004, kept that love alive, too. Thank you to Donna Raditic, D.V.M., who graciously read the entire original manuscript for medical accuracy and clarified many issues. I want to thank Lorraine Rosenthal of Cancer Control Society, who believed in this work and helped the second edition happen. Throughout the entire process from acceptance to final print to a revised edition, I have enjoyed working with the team at Healing Arts Press who are responsive, have a sense of humor, and remain fair to writers. My special thanks to acquisitions editor Jon Graham, sales associate/marketing editor Andy Raymond, my editor for this revised edition Jamaica Burns, and to Elaine Cissi for her work on the first edition.

Finally, I could not have written this book without the help of so many veterinarians, other animal care practitioners, animal lovers, and writers. Special thanks for help with this edition go to George Glanzberg,

Narda Robinson, Myrna Milani, Rita Reynolds, Marilyn Putz, Debra Theriault, Cynthia Otto, Stephanie LaFarge, W. Jean Dodds, Robert McDowell, Randy Grim, Susan Hamlin, Michael McFarland, Dale Moss, Andrea Spencer, and Charles K. Short. They were generous, kind, and instructive and were not bothered if I asked them questions that might have seemed elementary. I also thank each of them for all the continued, important work they do on behalf of animals.

Introduction

I am not a veterinarian, but I am a longtime journalist, an avid researcher and teacher of research techniques, and an animal lover. I have been writing about animal companions for more than a decade, have lived with them for the bulk of my fifty years, and, in the past twenty years, have lost four of them to four different types of cancer (one was feline leukemia, but may have involved another cancer at the end). I and my animals have not tried all the complementary methods of treatment listed in this book, but I am open-minded, and I wanted to include most of the available options. This book is not meant to endorse any one particular treatment but is intended instead to help you in your understanding and objective evaluation of the possible causes and variety of treatments for cancer in our animal companions.

Our knowledge of cancer keeps evolving. Lots of new treatments are currently being tested; herbal preparations and homeopathic remedies are being reconsidered; new genetic theories are being discussed. Keeping up in this field would be a full-time job. Then there is the sometimes overwhelming existence of the Internet; while a good source of information, it is also full of chat rooms and fly-by-night cures of which you should be cautious. Many animal Web sites are merely fan clubs or memorials to departed pets. I have no interest in presenting "cures" that do not work or getting anyone's hopes up for naught.

Our animals are living longer these days, and they are developing more cancers. We have, in our speed and efficiency, provided more and more ready-made products for them, but some of these are dangerous. We may often spend less time with our animal companions because we are just too busy. We may buy them the types of commercial food we can find most readily. We may be vaccinating them against a few virulent diseases, yet this increased number of vaccinations may be abetting or causing various cancers. We may be providing them with an old standby brand of cat litter or a popular chewy toy that may cause them serious damage. Even flea remedies and ordinary drinking water can hold risks. Are we loving our animals to death?

On the positive side, cancer continues to be big news, in humans and in animals. A huge amount of information bombards us almost every day from a variety of sources, both scholarly and popular. (One of the most surprising articles I found was printed in *Popular Mechanics*!) And some of the news about cutting-edge treatments, drugs, and herbal therapies for humans also pertains to animals or will in the very near future.

Throughout my work on this project, at least 90 percent of the veterinarians I contacted were forthcoming, generous, and kind. They were willing to share theories, case studies, or information with me—in spite of the fact that I was unknown to many of them—in the hope of saving or prolonging more domestic animals' lives.

That, too, is my intent. I wrote this book because animals have enriched my life and because I see our role regarding animals as that of stewards. We are entrusted with their well-being. I inherited from one of my mentors, Albert Schweitzer, a "reverence for all life."

The best way to avoid cancer in animals is to provide them with healthy lives—adequate exercise, appropriate medical attention, nutritious food, and lots of love. The more I research the topic, the more strongly I feel that prevention is the most critical way to avert or put off cancer. But if you already have an animal with cancer, it is wise to read as much as you can and to work with your primary veterinarian or other qualified health care professional first. Always find a veterinarian you feel you can trust implicitly, for both your and the animal's best interests. I do not recommend changing treatments or even diet without consulting one of these experts. Still, do not consider a diagnosis of cancer a death sentence; it needn't be. Each case is different, as is each animal. There is much more hope in treating many forms of cancer in dogs and cats, in particular, than there was fifteen years ago when our gray tiger cat, Misty, died of a mammary tumor.

I wish you well—and hope this book provides enough information to help your beloved animals enjoy a few more happy, pain-free, physically comfortable months or years with you.

1 Today's Pets, Today's Cancer

Recently, I traveled to Portland, Maine, with a couple visiting from Greece. Newlyweds in their early forties, they do not plan to have children. Trying to find a common bond, I asked the man if they had any animals. He said, "No. I had a dog when I was a child and then he died. Of course, it's natural. But it was so terrible. I couldn't live through that again."

Terrible is just what it is when your animal companion becomes ill and dies. You feel so helpless. Unlike children, who ultimately mature and become responsible for themselves, an animal requires your constant, life-long care. You are responsible for all aspects of her life. You hold her and comfort her, and you alter your daily routine to care for her. You cook her healthy meals and provide vitamins and minerals. Over the years you will probably watch her deteriorate, hobble around, and die in your arms. Animals are excellent patients. Few complain or even utter a sound. Their emotions are in their eyes. As they have always done, they trust that you will make the best decisions on their part.

I know how terrible the death of an animal companion is. In the past fifteen years four of our five domestic animals—three cats and a dog—have died of cancer or a related illness. One cat, Annie, died of feline leukemia (not considered a cancer in animals, but often associated with a secondary cancerous disorder or lymphoma) at eighteen; another, Misty, of mammary cancer, also at eighteen. Our dog Bauhaus died of a mast cell tumor in her neck at twelve, and the fourth, Puck, an eight-year-old cat, died of a vaccine-induced fibrosarcoma. Three of the animals had one or two surgeries and we made dietary changes, but we did not attempt chemotherapy or radiation primarily because of the cost and the distance we would have to travel. The experiences were wrenching. It is especially painful to see the ugly growths become larger and larger, something we seldom see in humans. Two of the only times I have seen my husband almost faint and actually cry were during the times of our pets' illnesses and deaths.

Unfortunately, our experiences are not uncommon. In preparation for this book I talked with friends, relatives, neighbors, colleagues, and animal care professionals. I was stunned to discover that each had an animal cancer story. In one day I heard of two dogs with leg or bone cancer, one three years old, the other eight. Both will undergo amputations and chemotherapy. The procedures are expensive, painful, and always traumatic. I heard of a cat who died of liver cancer at age fourteen. In a single year a colleague's dog and cat both died of cancer, even though he drove two hundred miles once a week so they could receive radiation treatments.

In a span of three days I learned of one cat, age eighteen, who died of cancer; another friend's elderly cat had a growth removed, which is being biopsied; and a growth has redeveloped on my cousin's dog's neck. The first was merely a cyst, but its recurrence is worrisome to someone like me because of our similar experiences with our own dog Bauhaus. These sad tales are not unusual once you start to pay attention.

While caring for our own ill animals, my resolve to take action grew stronger. As our animals continued to get sick, we made every effort we could to be certain we were providing the best and safest care for them. We had a tap water test done to check for lead; it came back negative. We don't smoke or use pesticides. We made dietary changes for our subsequent cats and dog. We no longer bought them any grocery store commercial foods, purchasing instead only high-quality "natural" foods at pet stores. I decided to do some research to see if other people were experiencing as many painful deaths as we were. I discovered that many people we knew had similar cancer stories to tell, although perhaps not so many in rapid succession. After looking for resources to learn more about cancer in animals and its prevention and treatment, and finding few available, I decided to write one. I determined to do everything I could to help other animals and their human companions avoid this pernicious disease, to diagnose it earlier, or to provide a better chance for survival after diagnosis.

According to an October 1997 Morris Animal Foundation survey, (no new statistics were available as of October 2004) cancer is the number one killer of dogs and cats, and the number one concern of animal guardians. At least 25 percent of dogs and cats die from cancer; in some veterinary practices, 40 percent of the patients have some form of cancer. In the Morris study, which surveyed 2,003 pet owners, the leading cause of nonaccidental death in dogs was cancer (at 47 percent). In cats the three leading nonaccidental causes of death are dental problems, urinary problems, and cancer, the last at 32 percent.[1] That survey also identified cancer as the leading cause of disease-related deaths in ferrets (33 percent), rabbits (28 percent), and birds (18 percent).[2] Other studies indicate that 45 percent of dogs over ten years of age die of cancer. Some seventy types of cancer have been identified in domestic animals.

THE CHANGING STATUS OF DOMESTIC ANIMALS

In this book, because of my respect for all creatures, I will primarily refer to dogs, cats, and other animals as our "animal companions" or to us as their "guardians." If I slip back into "pet" occasionally, please forgive me! Pet is still the most familiar term, but many animal advocates, including this one, now believe this implies the wrong type of relationship between the two species. The word guardian rather than owner is so much clearer and defines what our relationship with these creatures ought to be. According to Jan McHugh, Executive Director, Humane Society of Boulder Valley, quoted in a blurb for In Defense of Animals, an international animal protection organization, "Although it is a simple language change, we hope that the increased awareness of the 'guardian' language will elevate the status of animals in our community. We will use the word 'guardian' as another tool to fight animal abuse and exploitation."[3] In fact, as of August 2004, thirteen American cities, one county, and one entire state, Rhode Island, have passed legislation to change the wording of what were formerly known as "pet owners" to "animal guardians."[4]

Animals are critically important in our lives. For many, they are almost like children. They bring balance to lives often out of control in terms of speed and reliance on technology. They make us exercise regularly; they show us unconditional love. They lower our blood pressure; they understand when we have had a bad day. My dog Wanda eased the pain of my father's death. They make us laugh.

An increasing number of North Americans are living with animals, frequently with multiple animals. Because the numbers of pets are hard to count, statistics vary widely, but an estimated 60 million dogs and 70 million cats currently live in homes in the United States.[5]

The dog population is slightly decreasing, because dogs are more complicated to care for. Small animals, such as ferrets and hamsters, are rising in popularity because of their size and ease of care.[6] Turtles, snakes, and lizards are growing in popularity too. Birds living in U.S. households made two million visits to veterinarians in 2001.[7]

Nancy Peterson, an issues specialist with the Humane Society of the United States, describes our relationships with our animal companions eloquently: "The benefits of animal companionship are numerous. Pets serve as teachers and therapists and healers, friends and family, and without them our lives would be greatly diminished."[8] Especially for those without children, the lonely, and the elderly, these creatures are essential to well-being. Pets help children learn to communicate and to respect nature. They teach responsibility. For older people, pets provide companionship and love. Animals also make them feel safer, and often make them keep the heat higher, thus also keeping themselves warmer. Having a dog makes them exercise more. Pets in general can alleviate people's focusing inward on their own disabilities or problems and can provide distractions from depression, bereavement, or pain.[9] Just owning a pet that you can hold and stroke lowers blood pressure, reduces stress, and encourages better physical fitness. In Japan, if you don't live with an animal companion, commercial establishments exist that let you engage in ninety-minute sessions of patting and playing with a dog; five sessions cost $1,800.[10]

The Delta Society, a national nonprofit association in the field of human-animal interactions, recently compiled a list of reasons to live with an animal companion. Here are just a few of the group's findings: Seniors who own dogs go to the doctor less frequently. Animal guardians have lower triglyceride and cholesterol levels. Animal companions, especially dogs, help children adjust better to the serious illness or death of a parent. Animal guardians feel less afraid of crime when walking or living with a dog and have higher one-year survival rates following the onset of coronary heart disease. In nursing homes in New York, Missouri, and Texas, medication costs per patient per day dropped from $3.80 to $1.18 when animals and plants were part of the environment. These are only a few of the benefits of sharing our lives with animals.[11]

In a 1983 survey at Tufts University 80 percent of the 463 total respondents cited animal companions as a source of cheerfulness; 73 percent of total respondents considered them members of the family; 70 percent considered an animal companion a "thing of beauty." Seven percent considered them a nuisance, and 4 percent a financial burden. In another survey about animal guardians' concerns, 73 percent of the 463 respondents were most concerned about an animal companion getting hit by a car; 70 percent about an animal eating something toxic; and 68 percent about illness. Still another poll listed the following as the top reasons for having animal companions: for the sheer pleasure, 79 percent; to give love to the animal, 67 percent; to cheer the home, 64 percent; and to receive love from the animal, 63 percent.[12]

Another sign that animals are being taken more seriously in our lives and society is that Humane Society of the United States researchers recently announced that at least eighty-nine colleges or universities in North America currently offer courses focused on animal ethics and welfare issues. They estimate that approximately five thousand college students are now receiving such instruction. Leading the way was Colorado State University, which offered a course on animals and society in 1978.[13] In addition, animal rights law specialties are on the rise at the nation's law schools. Forty law schools now offer animal law classes, and an Animal Law Conference was held at Yale University in November 2004.[14]

Apparently, pets can also help with grades. A fascinating new study of two hundred respondents between the ages of seventeen and twenty-five revealed a correlation between having an animal companion and achieving high SAT scores and grade point averages. On average, scores were higher for pet owners than for nonowners; the more time the student spent with the animal, the better the scores he or she received.[15]

Because we realize their value, we are treating our animal companions better—providing doggie day care and better nutrition, establishing dog parks, purchasing pet health insurance, and more. We are using them in pet therapy with the elderly, with prisoners, with disabled youngsters; we know they help us stay healthier, both physically and emotionally. Horses and llamas help disabled children and adults learn physical dexterity and responsibility. Dogs help children with behavioral problems or with autism reach out and feel connected. Dogs and cats provide companionship for those dying of AIDS when many humans abandon them.

Another indication of their importance as family members, at least in the United States, is that more and more divorces include joint-custody arrangements for the animals. According to a recent article in the *New York Times*, Arthur I. Hirsch, a divorce lawyer, said that the issue of pet custody, whether joint or otherwise, comes up in one out of twenty divorces. Psychotherapist Stephanie LaFarge, based with the American Society for the Prevention of Cruelty to Animals (ASPCA) in New York City, saw ten couples in two years who arranged pet joint custody; she feels she will see a lot more. A recent Hollywood movie, *Dog Park*, released in September 1999, was based on just this subject.[16]

According to a 1998 article on Angell Memorial Animal Hospital in *Life* magazine, Americans spend $2.8 billion on veterinary care every year; the services available to animals are almost equivalent to those for humans. In 1998 it was reported that the typical dog owner spent $275 a year on medical care, but many said they were willing to pay at least $5,000 to extend an animal's life.[17]

In the United States alone, spending on our animal companions has reached an all time high. According to the American Pet Products Manufacturers Association (APPMA), a not-for-profit trade organization, spending has "doubled from $17 billion in 1994 [annually] to a projected $34.3 billion for 2004." Explained Bob Vetere, APPMA chief operating officer and managing director, "These spending figures reflect a change that has been occurring over the past decade of pets transitioning into the family." In 2004, American animal guardians were expected to spend $7.9 billion for supplies and over-the-counter medications and $8.3 billion for veterinarian care.[18]

Of course, it's not only we Americans who love our pets. Italians, for example, continue to be crazy over their domestic animals. A law recently enacted in the town of Recanati made drafty kennels, chains, and cramped conditions illegal for animal companions. In January 2000 Mayor Fabio Corvatta introduced sixteen regulations for animal guardians (especially for those who had cats and dogs). Guardians must take good medical care of all animal companions. Regular visits to the veterinarian and advice on diets are obligatory. Animal companions' living quarters must be at minimum 9.6 square yards and well lit, with adequate air and comfortable temperatures for the animals. Chaining a dog's collar is forbidden except on rare occasions. Dogs are allowed to enter most parks and gardens in the town.[19]

In Australia pets also reign supreme. According to the Royal New South Wales Canine Council Ltd. (RNSWCC), Australia's AKC, there are 182 dogs for every 1,000 Australians and every year 25,000 pure-bred dogs are registered with the RNSWCC. Australians spend $1.17 billion each year on their dogs and the dog food market alone is worth $560 million a year.[20]

The Australian Companion Animal Council states that because of relationships with animal companions the country's people saved more than $2.2 billion in human health expenditures in 1994–95. The animal guardians (as opposed to those without animals in the household) "typically visit the doctor less often and use less medication; . . . have lower cholesterol and lower blood pressure; . . . recover more quickly from illness and surgery; . . . deal better with stressful situations; . . . and are less likely to report feeling lonely."[21]

More recently, Japan is increasing its number of domestic animals. Sarah Hartwell, who works for U.K.'s Cats Protection and adopts and cares for older cats, has written extensively about cat care around the world. In "Cat Food Around the World," she states that the number of pets and pet-owning households in Japan are increasing each year, with "10 million pet dogs and 7 million pet cats. Approximately 30% of Japanese households (45.06 million) keep a cat or dog. . . . Animals provide a sense of companionship."[22]

CANCER AND OUR ANIMAL COMPANIONS

It would seem that our animals' health, too, would benefit from these relationships. Yet despite all the money, attention, and love we lavish on our animal companions, cancer in a variety of forms keeps rearing its ugly head. Why? And how can we make the best possible decisions for these creatures, our best friends—after all they do for us?

Incidence of Cancer

In the United States cancer now afflicts 1 in approximately 3.5 adults aged sixty to seventy-nine and 1 in 55 before the age of thirty-nine.[23] It is the number two killer of humans, after cardiovascular disease. In domestic fact, cancer's rise in occurrence came first among humans, but animals are no longer far behind. Some other species can get almost as many kinds of cancer as we can.

No breed-specific genetic alterations have been found that predispose certain breeds to develop cancers, but some breeds do acquire the disease a bit more commonly than others. See chapter 2 for a current list of these canine breeds. Among cats, there is a high incidence of cancers in the Siamese breed.[24]

Definition of Cancer

For a brief refresher course, let me define some basic terms related to this disease. One definition of *cancer* is: "A malignant growth of tissue tending to spread and associated with general ill health and progressive emaciation."[25] Healthy cells grow, divide, and replace themselves, which keeps the body in good physical repair. Cancerous cells do not develop normally, but they do multiply and divide. There is no apparent order to their replication; neither is it always certain when they will reproduce, if ever. Each type of cancer cell has its own course of development; most of the cells develop into a mass called a tumor. Of course, some of these tumors are benign (not cancerous). They may grow, but they remain confined to the tissue in which they arise. These can usually be removed surgically, and the patient, human or animal, experiences a full recovery.

The tumors to worry about are the malignant ones, those that spread and destroy surrounding tissues. The spreading process of cancer is called metastasis. Common sites for metastases are the lungs, liver, bones, and brain.[26] In veterinary textbook language tumors are not called cancerous but, rather, neoplasms. They are also referred to as tumors on occasion. Perhaps the word *cancer* is just too scary for many of us to use.

No one cause of cancer has yet been found for humans or animals. The disease often occurs because of genetic mutations, which may be caused by contact with certain substances we call carcinogens. Carcinogens activate a chain of biological events that lead to cancer, with its varied symptoms. The process can happen rapidly or may take several years. Some animals are more sensitive to carcinogens than others; many risks factors are still unknown.[27] Certainly we know that among people the risk of cancer increases with smoking, being exposed to certain pesticides or other carcinogenic substances, poor diet, and more. Environmental agents associated with cancer in humans include viruses, tobacco, food, radiation, chemicals, and pollution. While environment and diet appear to be important factors in some human cancers, heredity plays a relatively small role—except in a few cases, such as breast cancer. (Five to 20 percent of human breast cancer cases reflect evidence of a strong inherited predisposition.[28]) Of course, animals continue to be used in experimentation to determine causes and treatments for human and animal cancers and other diseases. Currently, for instance, research is being performed on some breeds of dogs to determine the relationship between lineage and cancer.

Some of the factors involved in the development of cancer in our domestic animals mirror those involved in human cancer. Others seem much more specific to animal cancer than to the disease in humans. These factors, in no particular order, appear to be: their lengthening life spans; their diets, especially when these are entirely commercial with no additional nutrients; perhaps their drinking water; high levels of stress; genetic factors, which play a role in some species; environmental agents such as pesticides and herbicides; secondhand smoke; and a variety of vaccines, some of which may not be necessary or for which the site of vaccination can be switched. This book will address these factors and others that may play into the development of an animal's compromised immune system or weakened state of health.

Let me stress that there seems to be no agreement about what exactly causes cancer in animals—this is an extremely complex disease with many varieties. Some veterinarians say it is entirely genetic; some think diet and lifestyle issues are key. Some believe it is mostly a function of increased age. According to the veterinarians at Hill's Pet Food, animals are living longer for many reasons, including a decline in often fatal infectious diseases, more effective drugs, improved diagnostics and technology, and better-educated and more committed animal guardians. Animal companions are now, in most countries, recognized members of society and families and, as such, receive better health care and improved nutrition, leading to longer lives.[29]

Common Types of Cancer in Animals, Especially in Dogs and Cats

The All-Care Animal Referral Center in California lists seven varieties of common cancers found in animal companions. The American Veterinary Medical Association adds a few others to this list.

+ *Abdominal Tumors:* These are quite common but difficult to diagnose early on. Abdominal enlargement and weight loss are signs of these types of tumors.
+ *Bone Tumors:* These are quite common in large dogs but rare in cats. The leg bones near the joints are the most common sites for these tumors. Lameness or swelling of the leg are early warning signs.
+ *Brain Tumors:* These may occur in both dogs and cats as primary or metastatic tumors.
+ *Canine Mammary Tumors:* These are the most common tumors found in female dogs, generally those that are older. If a dog is spayed prior to her second heat cycle, the risk decreases. Approximately half of all mammary canine tumors are malignant.
+ *Feline Mammary Tumors:* These are generally seen in older female cats; our cat Misty was about eighteen when her tumors appeared. They tend to grow and metastasize rapidly. According to the American Veterinary Medical Association, 50 percent of breast tumors in dogs and 85 percent in cats are malignant. Spaying or neutering at an early age greatly reduces the risk.[30]
+ *Head, Nose, and Neck Cancers:* Mouth cancer is common in dogs, but less so in cats. Because many of these swellings are malignant, early treatment is critical. Masses on the gums, bleeding, odor, or difficulty eating are warning signs. Nasal cancers may occur in both cats and dogs. Signs are bleeding from the nose, labored breathing, or facial swelling.
+ *Lymphosarcomas:* This is a cancer of the lymphatic system that

occurs mostly in middle-aged animals (in cats, around eight to ten years; in dogs, around six to eight years).

+ *Mast Cell Tumors of the Skin:* These are skin tumors seen in middle-aged and old dogs and in older cats. These tumors metastasize to lymph nodes. Our mixed-breed (yellow Lab type) dog, Bauhaus, developed this cancer in her neck at the age of eleven.

+ *Melanomas:* These are skin cancers. They are usually solitary, black-pigmented tumors, either benign or malignant, and hard to control. Most skin cancers in cats are malignant; in dogs, they often are benign.[31]

+ *Osteosarcomas:* These are bone cancers most often seen in large breeds of dogs. The tumors metastasize quickly.

+ *Testicular Tumors:* Tumors on the testicles are rare in cats, but common in dogs. They show up particularly in those with retained testes.[32]

See chapters 2 and 3 for more information on specific cancers in dogs and cats, respectively, and chapter 4 for those that can affect other small animal companions.

Warning Signs of Cancer

As is true with any behavioral or physical change in your animal companion, warning signs of tumors both benign and malignant should be checked out thoroughly and immediately by your trusted veterinarian. All experts in the animal health field say that early detection and prompt diagnosis and treatment of cancer will increase the chances of recovery, or at least of a longer, happier life for the animal.

Here are what the majority of veterinary sources consider to be the possible symptoms of cancer:

+ Any abnormal swelling or lump that keeps growing.
+ Nonhealing sores.
+ Weight loss for no apparent reason.
+ Loss of normal appetite.
+ Bleeding or unusual discharge from a body opening such as the nose or mouth.
+ A foul odor, especially from the mouth.

+ Difficulty eating or swallowing.
+ Loss of strength and disinterest in normal exercise.
+ Lameness or stiffness that continues.
+ Difficulty breathing, defecating, or urinating.
+ Any other change in behavior. For example, some case studies regarding bone cancers indicated that the dog or cat first started limping.[33]

Prevention and Early Detection

Prevention and early detection can make all the difference. Marion S. Lane and the staff of the Humane Society of the United States write that "your best offense in protecting your [pet] against serious illness is a good defense"—including regular visits to your veterinarian; spaying or neutering, which helps prevent diseases of the reproductive organs as well as overpopulation and abandonment of animal companions; screening exams that your veterinarian recommends, especially as your animal ages; and careful observation and prompt investigation of "anything out of the ordinary."[34] And according to Steven E. Crow, D.V.M., malignant tumors identified during regular exams are more likely to be cured "than cancers which are already causing clinical signs of illnesses."[35]

Dr. Crow, head oncologist at the Sacramento Animal Medical Group, Sacramento, California, adds that the likelihood of many animal cancers can be significantly reduced in at least three ways:

+ Spaying female dogs prior to their first heat. This reduces the risk of breast cancer to 0.5 percent. An ovariohysterectomy after one heat cycle or two or more estrous cycles reduces the risk of mammary carcinomas to 8 or 26 percent, respectively.
+ Neutering male dogs eliminates all testicular tumors and decreases the possibility of circumanal adenomas and adenocarcinomas.
+ People with white or light-pigmented cats should minimize their pets' exposure to sunlight—especially between 10 A.M. and 4 P.M.—to protect against squamous cell carcinomas of the eyelids, nose, and ears; owners of white dogs can use sunscreens (up to SPF 30) and avoid excessive sun exposure. This may reduce the prevalence of solar-induced cancers, such as basal cell carcinomas and squamous cell carcinomas, on these dogs' noses.[36]

With dogs, watch for growths in the mouth and on the dog's body. Check each mammary gland periodically, approximately once a month. With male dogs, especially those older than six years, palpate the testicles to see changes in size that could indicate a growth.[37]

Here are a few more tips, especially important for all older pets:

+ Make annual medical checkups. Geriatric animals should be checked at least twice a year. (For large animals, or those who get especially anxious and cagey before and during trips to the vet, it is wonderful if you can find a veterinarian who makes home visits.)
+ Keep your animal on a well-balanced, nutritious diet.
+ Try not to needlessly alter your animal's routines. Changes can bring on stress. Try to feed and walk at regularly scheduled times.
+ Before bringing in a new pet, consider your older pet's reactions. Many older dogs and cats enjoy younger ones, while some do not. You can create misery, and possibly even illness, if you force a new roommate on a set-in-her-ways animal.
+ Keep your pets clean. They like it, and they feel nicer to your touch.[38]
+ Touch your animals regularly to establish closeness and to detect any early lumps or abnormalities. This is an important part of the human-animal bond.
+ Keep the water dish washed and full of clean water.
+ Play with your animals on a regular basis. It's good for both of you.

Dealing with Cancer

One issue of importance when dealing with cancer, in your human companions or furry ones, is to get a second or even third opinion. At the 2004 North American Veterinary Conference, this opinion was stressed: "Different cancer types require different strategies for treatment. Explanation of treatment procedures, discussing risks, benefits, toxicity, and costs must be combined with client discussions regarding a realistic, and unbiased view of all treatment options available, and the animal's likely prognosis. Second, third, or even fourth opinions are sometimes necessary to provide optimal therapy for an individual patient."[39]

In traditional Western medicine, of course, doctors and nurses treat symptoms with a variety of techniques that have been proved to work, fully or at least partially, for varying lengths of time. In the case of cancer, surgery, chemotherapy, radiation, changes in diet, and other medications are among them. But holistic practitioners tend to look at the whole person or animal and make larger lifestyle changes—*before* disease strikes, if possible. Indeed, many experts believe that in both people and in animals, the best ways to treat cancer—to lessen its risks—are prevention and early detection.

Marion S. Lane and the staff of the Humane Society of the United States say it quite succinctly in *Complete Guide to Dog Care:* "There seems to be more evidence every day that we humans can help prevent disease and disability by exercising, eating well, and managing the stress in our lives. The same is true for our dogs [and cats, ferrets, and so forth], but in their case, we're the ones who are in control of their diet, their exercise, and their lifestyle . . . just start thinking about the fact that your focus on prevention can have a big impact on your dog's health and welfare."[40]

As Rachel Carson, author of *Silent Spring,* wrote in 1962: "Today we find our world filled with cancer-producing agents. An attack on cancer that is concentrated wholly or even largely on therapeutic measures . . . will fail because it leaves untouched the great reservoirs of carcinogenic agents which would continue to claim new victims faster than the as yet elusive 'cure' could allay the disease." She quotes W. C. Hueper, who said that "the goal of curing the victims of cancer is more exciting, more tangible, more glamorous and rewarding than prevention."[41]

These attitudes about "curing" still seem to abound even as the numbers of the sick climb. Much progress has been made, of course, with humans and now with domestic animals. But our world has more carcinogens, and many of us spend less time on diet or on exercise as we hurry, hurry, hurry to meet the increasing number of demands on our time. Pet food, for instance, was developed to help the busy housewife, yet many veterinarians and animal dietitians today believe that a homemade diet is ultimately better for our pets. I will discuss this in great detail later. Both the fight for cures and the attention paid to prevention must continue if we are to save more animals' lives.

As Carson also wrote, "For those in whom cancer is already a hidden or a visible presence, efforts to find cures must of course continue. But for those not yet touched by the disease and certainly for the generations as yet unborn, prevention is the imperative need."[42]

THREE COMPELLING THEORIES ABOUT THE CAUSES OF CANCER AND OTHER DISEASES

Myrna Milani, D.V.M., is a veterinarian in New Hampshire who, these days, does a lot of work with aggressive dogs and their guardians. "I have a primarily referral bond/behavioral practice, the bulk of which deals with behavioral problems, particularly aggression," she explains. Milani holds strong opinions, does her research, and has penned several excellent and provocative books about the animal-human bond. Although I have not seen this theory being discussed among other American veterinarians, she told me that vets in other countries have thought of this. She says that only the U.S. is so "obsessed with spaying and neutering," which to her is at the root of many problems. Here is what she has to say. I am including a rather long quote because she is so eloquent on her subject:

> When I looked at pet dogs and cats and asked what the major difference between them and their owners is, the politically incorrect answer was sterilization. Not only does it affect the individual, but also the species. On the individual level, there is a growing body of research on the nonreproductive effects of hormones and there is a whole science, psychoneuroimmunology, that explores the relationship between hormones, the immune response and the brain and central nervous system, all of which are intimately and inextricably connected. When we remove an animal's primary source of sex hormones, we may render them more susceptible to stress, and less capable of handling it. Attempts to handle it will stress other organs and undermine the immune response that then could predispose the animal to immune-mediated problems, including cancer.
>
> On the species front, if all the responsible owners spay and neuter their pets, who determines the make-up of the canine gene

pool? We are increasingly dependent on a canine gene pool coming from the worst sources (relative to the needs of the pet animal
owner population) at the same time that we are demanding our
pets fulfill ever more complex human emotional needs. Even
though the party line has always been that it's those who don't care
enough who are destroying companion animals, I think you could
make a very good case that those who care/love too much create
as many problems for them.

Milani points to various studies on related issues: "One study has
shown a link between osteosarcoma (bone cancer) and early neutering
in rottweilers, so delving into the reason for all these cancers (both dogs
and cats are more likely to die of them than humans) may mean taking
a hard look at some aspects of pet ownership we'd rather not consider"
(i.e., our responsibilities, spaying and neutering, love and what it
means).

Milani is somewhat more concerned with dogs' overall health,
because they are more dependent on us as their guardians. "Cats are suf-
ficiently undomesticated that they can escape and make it on their own.
Still, they are caught on that thin line between buying into a dependent
relationship with us or going it alone and that's got to be stressful. Given
the role of the thyroid in the immune response, it's interesting that our
least domesticated species succumbs to hyperthyroidism whereas our
most falls prey to hypothyroidism. My guess is that cats will probably fall
victim to hypothyroidism, too, as time goes on."[43]

Alfred J. Plechner, D.V.M., has been a successful veterinarian for thirty-
six years. He currently practices in West Los Angeles. Throughout the
process of seeing more than 50,000 patients over the years, and seeing
patterns of recurring illnesses, he came to recognize that "devastating
endrocrine-immune imbalances result from an unsuspected deficiency
or defect in cortisol, an important adrenal hormonal."[44] He tests for
this deficiency and then administers very low dosages of cortisone on a
long-term basis. He uses both synthetic cortisone and a natural cortisol
preparation and stresses that at low dosages, they are "significant healing agents for many seemingly unrelated diseases," including allergies,
obesity, autoimmune disorders, food hypersensitivity, aggressiveness,

and cancer. This treatment also works for "animals unresponsive to conventional treatment," he writes in his eye-opening book, *Pets At Risk* (NewSage Press, 2003), written, with Martin Zucker, for both veterinarians and for animal guardians. The team's first book was *Pet Allergies.*

Plechner explains that animals with such endocrine-immune imbalances usually recover quickly. "However, you cannot stop the program once you see improvement and recovery. The program I have developed compensates for a physiological deficiency with medication that acts as a hormone replacement." His treatment includes both the cortisone and a "diet that does not contain offending foods."[45]

As do many open-minded veterinarians, Plechner also links adrenal dysfunction to food allergies, environmental causes, and stress. And he believes that the animal guardian is crucial in all healing. "The animal's guardian and the animal's doctor must form a congenial partnership. . . . There are things that only a veterinarian can do, and there are things that only a pet owner can do," he states.[46]

In my research, I have always found the Australians to be more open-minded and alternative medicine-minded than most Americans. When I found herbalist Robert McDowell, N.D., who lives in Bathurst, Australia, near Dr. Ian Billinghurst (see B.A.R.F. diet in nutrition chapter), I found yet another theory that deserves inclusion. Although McDowell sells herbal treatments, he also treats individual dogs and has several years experience dealing with cancer.

Here is what he believes is at the root of the increase in cancer, at least among dogs: "There seems to be a cruel parallel between the rise in the incidence of Canine Cancers and the same trend in Human Cancers. . . . In the case of domesticated dogs, Cancer is on the rise, developmental disorders are commonplace, life expectancy is shortening and domestic dogs are more fragile and more expensive to maintain nowadays, than ever before." Why is this happening, we might ask? According to McDowell, the wrong lifestyle, in a nutshell. We are feeding our dogs poorly and not providing adequate exercise. "We are subverting our dog's environment along with our own, by introducing stress, boredom, snack foods, overeating, poor exercise patterns, artificial lighting and over-medication, to name a few." McDowell feels that the two primary factors in the increase in cancer rates are "Our canine companions' 'modern diet,' and subverted exercise patterns."

He recommends Dr. Billinghurst's B.A.R.F. diet, an acronym for Bones and Raw Food, especially "meat, offal and bones, eggs, millet and linseed, green and root vegetables, wheat germ, cod liver oil, kelp and a small amount of table scraps." He would also recommend a bit of garlic, some dandelion, comfrey, and "the odd exposure to Rosehips."[47] Finally, overall, he wants us to treat our dogs in a more natural, fun way. "Enjoy, and let your pet enjoy, the health and improvement that flow from this. Don't give your dog any 'treats' other than raw meaty bones and space to run freely in."

Although he also treats cats and horses, he does not have as much data on cancer in these species. However, he writes me, "I treated very few equine or feline cancers (apart from melanomas in horses) up until the past three or four years and now the variety and frequency seems to be increasing which is to me, clear evidence that we are following the same course with these species as well." Horses need "a little green pick" and cats need "to escape and catch its [their] own prey at times. This saves them, perhaps, a little."[48]

2 Dogs

The two most popular domestic companions continue to be dogs and cats. Of these two species, dogs suffer from a considerably higher incidence of cancer.

Dogs live with people all over the world. We have lived in close contact with them for more than fifteen thousand years. This is the species most adapted to living easily with humans. Currently, almost fifty-six million dogs live with U.S. families; 38 percent of all households in this country include one dog. However, this number has decreased steadily since 1981, when more than 44 percent of households shared their space with at least one dog. Most dog people currently have one dog, but one in ten guardians lives with three or more canines.[1] According to statistics from the American Veterinary Medical Association, in the United States alone there are more than 7.3 million dogs aged eleven or older; this represents approximately 14 percent of dogs in this country.[2] In another country wild for dogs, Australia, 37 percent of all households live with at least one dog.[3]

Dogs come in a remarkable variety of shapes and sizes. The American Kennel Club (AKC), that elite purebred association founded about 110 years ago, currently recognizes 153 breeds, but *The Atlas of Dog Breeds of the World* by Bonnie Wilcox, D.V.M., and Chris Walkowicz lists more than 400 breeds, while *Simon & Schuster's Guide to Dogs* lists 320 breeds.

Dogs have shorter lives than cats. Generally, a dog's life span ranges from eight to fifteen years, with smaller dogs often living the longest. In a study of 23,535 deceased dogs obtained from a computerized database of North American veterinary teaching hospitals, researchers found that body size in the dog was inversely related to longevity. Also, the median age at death was considerably lower for purebred dogs than for mixed-breed dogs within each body weight group.[4] Supposedly, the longest-lived dog ever was an Australian cattle dog who lived to be an incredible twenty-nine years old![5]

Dogs make almost ideal companions. As Randy Grim, the man who saves urban street dogs, says in the book about his work, *The Man Who Talks to Dogs,* "They tell you when they're hungry, when they're sad, when they're happy. I mean, they're just like us; they're living, breathing beings who search for happiness just like we do. They want comfort. They want a nice place to sleep, good food, and treats. They want to be loved and wanted."[6]

Of course, cancer is not the only disease that canines share with humans. According to Nathan B. Sutter and Elaine A. Ostrander, "the top ten diseases in purebred dogs include several that are of concern to human health, such as cancer, epilepsy, autoimmune diseases, blindness, cataracts and heart disease."[7]

CANCERS

According to a Morris Animal Foundation survey, cancer is the number one killer of dogs and cats, at 47 percent, and the number one concern of animal guardians. The foundation lists the most common canine cancers as skin tumors, breast cancers, lymphomas, and cancers of the mouth and nose.[8] A few canine breeds seem to develop cancer more frequently than others. According to the American Kennel Club Canine Health Foundation, these are the Airedale terrier, akita, American Eskimo dog, Belgian malinois, bloodhound, boxer, briard, Canaan dog, curly-coated retriever, Dandie Dinmont terrier, English foxhound, English setter, flat-coated retriever, German wirehaired pointer, Great Dane, greyhound, Irish water spaniel, Irish wolfhound, Japanese chin, kuvasz, otterhound, Pembroke Welsh corgi, Portuguese water dog, Rhodesian ridgeback, rottweiler, Scottish deerhound, Scottish terrier, Skye terrier, soft-coated wheaten terrier, Staffordshire terrier, Tibetan terrier, and vizsla. This number, thirty-two, is up from twenty-one in 2002, with a few additions and deletions.[9]

But not all dogs that seem to acquire the disease are on this list. For example, of late, the Irish setter has seen a rise in cancers. In a health survey completed by the Irish Setter Club of America with the help of Purdue University in 1997, neoplasia was the most common cause of death. Among 436 Irish setters, 146 died of cancer. The most common type was breast cancer, affecting thirty dogs. An earlier survey of members, in 1992, showed that of 356 respondents, 43 percent reported an incidence of cancer in their dogs.[10]

In another study, as part of work being done to create a complete canine genome, researchers have linked kidney cancer to German shepherds. "Many of the same cancers that occur in humans are observed at a very high frequency in certain dog breeds. Breed-associated cancers are observed for Boxers and Pointers (lymphoma), Airedale Terriers and Golden Retrievers (soft tissue tumors), Scottish Terriers (melanoma), Scottish Deerhounds and Rotweillers (osteosarcoma) and Sky[e] Terriers (breast cancer). . . . We hypothesize that genes involved in both human and canine cancer biology can be mapped," write Frode Lingaas et al., in their paper about multifocal renal cystadenocarcinoma and nodular dermatofibrosis in the German shepherd dog.[11]

Breeds with generally low rates of cancer include the beagle, poodle, collie, and dachshund. The high rate of cancer in breeds such as the cocker spaniel and boxer has been linked to their great popularity and active breeding in the 1940s and 1950s.[12]

Large breeds are often susceptible to bone cancers. Black dogs often develop more melanoma cancers; oral melanoma is frequently found in dogs that have dark pigmentation in their mouths, such as German shepherds or cocker spaniels.[13] Unspayed female dogs or those spayed later in life may acquire mammary gland cancer, and unneutered male dogs may risk testicular cancer.[14] Spaying and neutering are advisable for a number of reasons, including lowering the probability of the latter two diseases. (See the end of chapter one, Dr. Myrna Milani's theory, for another viewpoint on this.)

As dogs age, they develop more cancers and other age-related diseases. According to several sources, some of the most common tumors include skin cancers, breast tumors, and osteogenic sarcomas, or bone cancers. Skin cancers include the following:

+ *Mast cell tumors* are common in older dogs and quite prevalent in certain breeds. About one-third of these are malignant.

According to Dr. Rodney Page, D.V.M., director of the Comparative Cancer Program at Cornell University's College of Veterinary Medicine, this is one malignant skin tumor that is frequently seen. It is "a common cancer that most veterinarians will see at some point during their careers. Mast cells are essentially white blood cells that respond to allergic conditions under normal circumstances." They are found only in dogs, in skin and other tissues, such as cartilage and bone. Golden retrievers and Labrador retrievers often acquire these tumors, as do Boxers.[15]

+ *Epidermoid carcinomas* are cauliflower-like tumors or hard ulcers that do not heal. They usually occur on the feet and legs.

+ *Melanomas* are often malignant neoplasms, dark in color. These may first appear to be only moles, but if they spread, bleed, or become elevated, they are probably melanomas. Cocker spaniels, Boston terriers, and Scottish terriers are a few breeds affected by this type of cancer.[16] According to Mike Richards, D.V.M., most malignant melanomas occur on the toes or in the mouth.[17]

Breast tumors are the most common cancer in dogs; they represent 52 percent of dog tumors. However, their numbers have declined over the past several years, according to Robert Runyan, D.V.M., because more dogs are being spayed at younger ages. Runyan says that dogs spayed before their first heat—at three months or so—have a 5 percent chance of growing mammary tumors. Dogs spayed after their first heat have a much higher risk: 26 percent.[18] (However, early spaying is somewhat controversial; some animal rights advocates feel the procedure is far too intrusive for a puppy of only three months of age.)

About half of mammary tumors are malignant. They may spread, especially to the lungs. Dr. Runyan believes that they ought to be surgically removed; if this is not done, tumors will continue to grow, eventually opening and draining "blood-tinged" fluid. The dog may have increased difficulty with her breathing as the tumors grow into her lungs. Runyan says that this cancer can be cured by "early, aggressive removal," but that chemotherapy or radiation therapy is not generally effective.[19] While male dogs can get mammary tumors, it is, as for human males, extremely rare.

Osteogenic sarcomas (bone cancers) appear on the long bones of the legs or the flat bones of the ribs, generally in middle-aged dogs. More males than females get this type of cancer; large breeds are particularly susceptible.[20] Amputations are sometimes necessary; see the success stories in chapter 17.

As of this new edition, a treatment for this type of cancer has emerged so that amputation is not always necessary. In some cases, doctors may do a limb-sparing surgery, using chemotherapy. According to Stephen J. Withrow, D.V.M., "the rate of local recurrence of osteosarcoma after limb-sparing surgery in dogs and humans has been reported up to 28%." He performed a study to look at whether a biodegradable cisplatin (a clear fluid type of chemotherapy) containing implant, inserted into the limb area at the time of surgery, would decrease the rate of local recurrence of the tumor. For his study, he looked at eighty dogs who had "spontaneously occurring osteosarcoma" and treated them with limb-sparing surgery. Some received the biodegradable implant with cisplatin and others received no cisplatin. Withrow's results showed that the group who received the chemotherapy in the form of cisplatin was "53.5% less likely to develop local recurrence than dogs in the control group." His conclusion states that "local tumor recurrence may be decreased . . ." so he is cautiously optimistic about his findings.[21]

Lymphoma is another common cancer in dogs and its incidence appears to be rising. It generally has its onset in middle age. Airedales, Basset hounds, Boxers, Bulldogs, St. Bernards, Bull mastiffs, and Scottish terriers seem to have an increased risk.[22] A brief remission of approximately eight to ten months is possible, but there is no known scientific cure. Scientists have found that a major barrier to treating lymphoma is its drug resistance. Most dogs with lymphoma do respond well to chemotherapy; remission rates with such therapy stand at approximately 80 to 90 percent. What happens, however, is that within a year most of these dogs become resistant to the drug and suffer a relapse. Researchers are currently addressing this issue in the hope of finding more effective treatments for lymphoma.[23]

Two diagnostic tests for lymphomas are needle aspirates, which study a small sample of cells literally sucked out of the lymph node and smeared onto a slide, and Tru-Cut biopsies, which examine a small core of lymph node that involves more tissue area than the needle aspirate, but less than an entire node surgical biopsy. This latter treatment can be done with a local anesthetic in most instances,[24] though this depends entirely on each specific patient.

While many of the cancers dogs acquire—including those you can neither see nor feel in a dog's body—cause her metabolism to behave abnormally throughout her life, a recent study from the nonprofit Morris Animal Foundation suggests that with comprehensive care (diet, surgery, and/or chemotherapy) a dog with cancer may live up to three years, and possibly longer.[25]

The depression of the normal immune response in older dogs might help explain, in part, the higher incidence of cancer in older animals.[26] Cancer is most often a disease of older age. One theory is that as cells divide throughout life, there occurs an increased chance of genetic mutation due to cell division "accidents" and to the accumulated effect of carcinogens. However, more than twenty inborn diseases in dogs are traced to defective genes; in all cases, the same defective gene has been found in humans. Dogs can even carry the braca 1 gene, identified as critical to a higher risk of breast cancer in women. Both the National Institutes of Health and the American Cancer Society have begun to fund the study of canine genetics because of its similarity to human genetic-based disease research.[27]

Obesity can increase the risk of cancer in dogs as well as lead to other ailments. Some reports indicate that the incidence of potential reproduction problems is 64 percent higher in overweight dogs than in others. An overweight dog also carries an increased surgical and anesthetic risk, because fat alters drug kinetics, may have an influence on anesthesia management, and may lower pulmonary function.[28]

Of course, as is true with all household animals, it is important to keep a close watch on your dog's body, mood, energy level, and eating and bathroom habits. Massage or pet your dog often for the good of your relationship and also to feel if any lumps or bumps have appeared. If a tumor begins in an internal organ, a lump will not be visible. It is advisable to have a veterinarian check any new growth to determine if it requires further investigation. Some of the further checks a veterinarian may perform include abdominal palpation, X-rays, ultrasounds, and routine blood tests.

TVT—Transmissible Venereal Tumor

Transmissible Venereal Tumor (TVT), known for many years but not often seen by most veterinarians, is most commonly found in dogs that live in packs, i.e., urban street dogs, many of whom have never lived with people. Randy Grim, subject of the book, *The Man Who Talks to Dogs,* who runs Stray Rescue of St. Louis for this population of dogs in Missouri, says that over the past five years he has seen this cancer increasing. "Up to seventy-five percent of the dogs we see from East Saint Louis have this cancer. [He sees far fewer from Saint Louis proper. In East Saint Louis, there are larger packs and no animal control.] They are not neutered, and when they give birth to pups, they can transmit it."[29]

Grim has been noticing this form of cancer for five years. It displays itself quite prominently as either "a big tumor sticking out of the vagina or dripping blood out of the dog's penis." "Surgery and six weeks of chemotherapy seem to treat most of the dogs," he allows. "So, in 2003, we captured 2,000 dogs. More than 1,000 of those had TVT. I wonder how many went un-diagnosed years ago, and if this is a problem in the puppy mills?"[30]

One of the veterinarians who treats Grim's dogs is Dr. Ed Migneco, D.V.M., owner of Hillside Animal Hospital (formerly City Animal Hospital) in St. Louis. He has treated almost nine hundred dogs for Grim and also helps other nonprofit groups with their animal needs. He admits that the number of dogs he sees with TVT is extremely high, but only in homeless urban dogs. It is transmitted by sexual behavior. He has only seen one case in an unneutered female domestic companion animal. "But it is one of the absolutely curable forms of cancer with relatively simple chemotherapy. The drug is Vincristine. It is given intravenously, one time a week, from six weeks to 12 weeks. Sometimes, even in two weeks, the tumor will shrink." The tumors occur both inside and outside the dog, sometimes even developing "inside and protruding to the outside." Unfortunately, two of Randy's dogs developed a malignant form of this cancer, but explains Dr. Migneco, "This is extremely unusual. The pathologist had never seen this before."[31]

OTHER LUMPS

Of course, many lumps—including cysts, warts, sebaceous cysts, papillomas, lipomas, and hematomas—are noncancerous. Hematomas often disappear by themselves, but the others can be drained (depending on the health of the animal—especially if draining requires general anesthetic), removed, or kept under a watchful eye, especially if they start to bleed. Still, these are not malignant and will not require as extensive a treatment protocol as the more harmful, sometimes life-threatening malignant growths.

Three other types of nonmalignant growths are ear flap hematomas, often due to irritation from ear mites or infections; histiocytomas on the face, feet, or ears of younger dogs; and perianal gland tumors, which affect mostly males and can cause pain and become infected.[32]

THE HEROIC DOGS OF 9/11—A SPECIAL CASE

When the World Trade Center (WTC) and the Pentagon were attacked on September 11, 2001, it was not only humans who worked for days, weeks, even months to find survivors or victims amongst the rubble. More than one hundred dogs, trained by FEMA (the Federal Emergency Management Agency) and others, worked at the World Trade Center and elsewhere untiringly and willingly to search out whatever hope they could find for loved ones who remained. The dogs were a variety of breeds, including German shepherds, Australian shepherds, all three varieties of Labrador retrievers, Doberman pincers, border collies, and many others including "pound puppies."[33]

Because of the amount of debris and toxins in the air, and because of the extremely stressful work (looking for bodies and often finding them already dead), several dog advocates (including this author) have worried about the physical and psychological outcomes for these dogs. Indeed, so far, fourteen have since died.

Since the attacks, a team of researchers at the University of Pennsylvania School of Veterinary Medicine has been monitoring the health of ninety-seven of the deployed dogs who worked at Ground Zero, the Pentagon, and the Fresh Kills landfill on Staten Island, where the human debris from the WTC was taken. Several foundations—including AKC Canine Health Foundation, Veterinary Pet Insurance Co., and the Geraldine R. Dodge Foundation—contributed to the support of the study. As of October 2004, the AKC Canine Health foundation had just refunded the project for at least two more years, states Cynthia Otto, D.V.M., the study's lead researcher.

As the dogs live all over the country, the researchers rely on their veterinarians to obtain samples and X-rays for them to study.[34] Initially after the attacks, the researchers did find "significantly higher" antibodies in these search and rescue dogs. But, according to Dr. Otto, "We can't find any link at this point that ties the 14 deaths to events of Sept. 11. Some have passed away, but the causes of death are no different than in the control group. That is good news."[35]

Ten of the total dogs have developed some form of cancer, and nine of those have died. Otto explains the situation more fully: "The dogs have had osteosarcoma, hepatocellular carcinoma (liver cancer), renal carcinoma, neurofibroma (nerve sheath tumor), hemangiosarcoma, multiple myeloma and melanoma. . . . The average age of the nine dogs that died of cancer was nine years; the range was between six and 13 years."[36] Otto continues, "Given the mature age of these dogs and their expected lifespan, the few deaths that did occur were not statistically significant."[37]

Although one goal of the study is to ascertain if there is a definite link between the work and environmental factors and cancer, Otto explains, "At this point in the study [October 2004], we cannot prove any connection. It will take several more years of this study to determine if the exposure to hazardous materials at the disaster sites can be linked to the development of cancer in these dogs. Currently, though, we have found no statistical correlation between their exposure during deployment and the development of cancer."[38]

OTHER HAZARDS FOR DOGS

Overpopulation

Cancer is not the only problem facing today's pet dogs. The early twenty-first century is not an especially charmed time for them, even though it appears, in most Western societies, that we are spoiling them more than previous generations did. Dogs often seem to have cushy lives. However, while more of us are coming to realize their value in our lives, two other major problems exist in the world of dogs. The first is that there are just too many of them, in almost every country. Neutering and spaying are not practiced or encouraged enough; millions of dogs are killed in shelters annually throughout the United States and elsewhere. In underdeveloped countries perhaps millions of dogs wander without homes, and here in the United States approximately eight million cats and dogs a year are euthanized because they do not have homes. Shelters are full of dogs discarded through no fault of their own but, rather, because their guardians could not find the time or patience to include them in their stressed, overbusy lives.

The entire issue of neutering and spaying has become more complex, however. It seems our American society always wants quicker and quicker fixes, for everything, even medical matters. In 2004, the first chemical sterilant for puppies became available on the U.S. market. Neutersol, made up of zinc gluconate, neutralized by argenine, can be administered directly into the testicles of dogs, only those from three to ten months old. It was tested and approved by the FDA.

The product has been in the works since 1982, developed by the late Dr. Mostafa Fahim, of the University of Missouri-Columbia School of Medicine. However, according to Dr. Melanie Berson, director of the Division of Therapeutic Drugs for Non-Food Animals, FDA/Center for Veterinary Medicine, "unlike surgical castration, dogs treated with Neutersol become sterile without removal of the testicles and, therefore, testosterone is not completely eliminated. Testosterone-related diseases, such as prostate disease and tumors located near the testicles and anus, may not be prevented with this procedure. As with surgical castration, secondary male characteristics (roaming, marking, aggression, or mounting) may still occur."[39]

A related drug, Suprelorin, has been approved in Australia for use on male dogs. This drug "focuses on regulating GnRH or Gonadatropin-releasing hormones," writes Joyce Briggs for the magazine, *Paws to Think*. Produced by Peptech Animal Health, it is marketed for "temporary control of fertility" and requires repeat visits to the local veterinarian.[40]

If you decide to neuter your male dog, research these products carefully. Several consumers and animal protection groups are opposed to Neutersol and at least one veterinarian I spoke with is not convinced enough to use the technique on his dogs. Explained Dr. Ed Migneco, D.V.M., "I have not had any personal experience with Neutersol. I have some reservations about it, though. Supposedly the dogs still have a small amount of testosterone produced. So, I wonder how will this affect the possibility of prostate enlargement, which is very common in unneutered male dogs? And will these dogs still act like intact males? I don't have the answers to these questions, so right now I am not a proponent of this technique."[41]

Genetic Problems

Many dogs and breeds are in worse genetic condition and general health than ever before. The genetic situation is a huge problem in the United States, Canada, Western Europe, Australia, England, and other countries where dog breeding is extremely serious business.

The domestic dogs of fifty years ago were healthier than the dogs of today, with fewer diseases and fewer afflictions specific to breed. A century ago most dogs were bred for functions—hunting, working, guarding, or being dependable companions. After World War II, however, breeders began to shift their emphasis to producing dogs that looked beautiful. The demand for beauty often superseded qualities such as intelligence, disposition, and genetic health. Line breeding—mating a dog to its granddam or grandsire—is practiced by some breeders. Inbreeding, mating a daughter to her father or a son to his mother (what we would call incest, which would produce devastating mental and physical problems in humans), is also a regular practice.

Since the 1950s veterinarians have noticed a higher percentage of dogs with genetically inherited problems. According to a recent *Time* magazine article, as many as 25 percent of purebred dogs in the United States have some genetic defect. Many breeds have even higher percentages. Hip dysplasia cripples many breeds. Eye, heart, and skin problems affect others. Little Pekinese dogs, a very old breed, often now have breathing difficulties, tooth loss, and inguinal hernias; their eyes could literally be knocked out of their recessed sockets if they took a steep fall.[42] The bulldog and Boston terrier have trouble whelping naturally because of their large heads. These bitches regularly must deliver by cesarean section. According to dog writer Mark Derr, more than three hundred genetic defects can affect dogs; no breeds are exempt. A number of studies have indicated that 15 to 30 percent of purebred puppies die before they are weaned. The more inbred they are, the higher the mortality rate. This is called fading puppy syndrome; no genetic component has yet been determined.[43]

Mixed breeds, those dogs not accepted by dog clubs or by most dog shows, are frequently healthier, have smoother dispositions, are more intelligent, and live longer than purebred dogs, although they do carry some genetic problems of their own. Writer Gary F. Mason has stated that more than five hundred genetic diseases have been identified in purebreds and more than one hundred in mutts.[44] And of course, if you adopt a mixed-breed dog, you have no idea of her parentage; her looks at adulthood may surprise you. (The result is often charming, as we discovered with our dog Wanda the Bearded Lady. As near as we can tell she is part Irish wolfhound, part black Lab, and part a few secret transients.)

Along with producing physical problems, excessive and often inappropriate breeding has affected the temperament of many breeds. Cocker spaniels, once extremely sweet, can now become snappy or antisocial. Sometimes golden retrievers can also become snappy, as can the huge Newfoundland. Puppy mills still churn out approximately half a million pups a year that fit a certain beauty standard but may not be friendly and may have serious genetic defects. (The pups are also raised in mostly substandard, often filthy conditions.)

By some estimates, up to 20 percent of today's domestic dogs display what owners and others consider behavior problems—including aggression, various phobias, and separation anxiety. These may result from one or more factors, including genetics, lifestyle issues, guardian neglect, and guardian misunderstanding or ignorance regarding normal canine behavior. Writes Mark Derr, author of *Dog's Best Friend: Annals of the Dog-Human Relationship*, "It [inbreeding] must be leavened with outcrosses to ensure the animals' genetic vitality and working ability . . . purity of bloodlines and uniform appearance are the least desirable characteristics one should seek in a breed." Derr adds that what is important to the AKC is beauty. "The standards do not demand that a dog be able to perform its traditional function—that the

Chesapeake be able to swim and fetch, for example."[45] Instead, what ought to be important in a canine are temperament, sound health, working ability, and what Derr labels basic "dogness,"[46] or those distinct habits, personality traits, and characteristics of the species.

According to Dug Hanbicki, issues specialist for animal companions for the Humane Society of the United States, 90 percent of the dogs sold in pet shops are produced in puppy mills, mostly found in the Midwest.[47] And the California Assembly Office of Research reported in 1998 that 48 percent of that state's pet store puppies were ill or recovering from an illness when they were purchased.[48]

As of December 2004, the Humane Society and other animal groups were still vigorously working against puppy mills. "The documented problems of puppy mills include overbreeding, inbreeding, minimal veterinary care, poor quality of food and shelter, lack of socialization with humans, overcrowded cages, and the killing of unwanted animals." The Humane Society of the United States estimates the number of puppies sold each year through pet stores to be approximately 500,000.[49]

Despite some genetic problems in purebred pups, many breeders work hard to maintain, even improve, their breed's health. Marilyn Putz of Highland Park, Illinois, is an Irish setter breeder who has lost five dogs to various cancers. "I have had setters since I was a child, and have always loved the breed. My five dogs who were cancer victims were not all related. I have been working closely in my breeding program with a friend who is also a breeder, and health is our first consideration, temperament, adherence to traits for which the breed was developed, and looks follow, in that order. We, and the Irish Setter Club of America's Health Committee, work very, very hard to improve the various breed problems, and have been quite successful in several instances," she told me. Although some critics worry about AKC standards placed on these dogs, Putz added, "Their major concern is the development and improvement of facets in breeds which promote the original purposes of specific breeds. This, of course, includes appearance . . . Of course, there are breeders who do not consider these factors, and breed just for appearances. It's my understanding that these people are becoming the minority, and that dog show judges are looking past superficial appearances. I hope that this is true."[50]

CANINE GENETICS AND CANCER RESEARCH

On the plus side for dogs, several universities and institutions are conducting genetics and cancer research on canines. The Morris Animal Foundation of Colorado, for instance, a fifty-six-year-old nonprofit organization founded to study small-animal health and fund animal health studies throughout the world, has sponsored more than 1,150 animal health studies with funds exceeding $36 million. "One hundred percent of all annual, unrestricted contributions support animal health studies, not administration or the cost of fund raising."[51]

Although veterinary scientists at universities study many health issues, cancer remains one of their largest areas of concern. Morris has been doing cancer-related studies since 1962; their first cancer study was for dogs. These studies could fill a book by themselves, but the following few are representative of the work being done on the conventional treatments of cancer.

Currently, Morris is funding studies on these canine cancer issues: osteosarcoma, mammary carcinoma, canine lesions, canine tumor tissue, canine squamous cell carcinoma, canine hemangiosarcoma, relapsed lymphoma in dogs, a study of Docetaxel, (a chemotherapeutic agent), another on canine lymphoma, osteosarcoma in Scottish deerhounds, two more regarding osteosarcoma, and another on mammary gland carcinoma.[52]

For an animal to be eligible for a study, explains Heidi Jeter, publications and media specialist, pet guardians need to contact the university where the study is taking place. "Investigators conducting clinical trials may be looking for participants and will have their own screening process. In general, animals can participate only in the clinical trials, so for example, most of the genetics studies are not done using live animals whereas a study testing a drug or treatment may be looking for participants." The animals usually require monitoring or follow-up visits throughout the period of study, so most interested parties need to live fairly close to that particular university.[53]

For some animals, enrollment in these studies can mean a longer, better life. One example is Aspen, a six-year-old female rottweiler diagnosed with bone cancer in July 1998. Her owner, Kurt Milliken of Colorado Springs, Colorado, was told that his dog would only live two to three months without surgery, three to four months if her leg was amputated, and maybe up to a year if he offered her combined amputation and chemotherapy. Probably the cancer would spread to her lungs, which would kill her.

What choice did he have? Following amputation and chemotherapy for Aspen, her veterinarian placed her in a study funded by the Morris Animal Foundation. That first study did not work for Aspen. Says Milliken, "Either Aspen got a placebo or the drug didn't work, because two days before Christmas, she was diagnosed with cancer in her lungs." But they did not give up on the dog. She then became enrolled in another Morris study centered on gene therapy. Her owner drove her to the hospital every day for six weeks; then every other week for twelve weeks; and finally, once a month.[54] As of October 1999 Aspen had been in remission for almost a year. Unfortunately, I don't know the end of this "success" story.

The AKC has done several dog-related cancer studies for many years. In November 2004, ten such studies were complete; ten were pending, i.e., looking for sponsors; and seventeen were active. Researchers are either Ph.D.'s or D.V.M.'s in states and provinces throughout North America. Various breed clubs, "random individuals" interested in specific breeds, or, in one instance, The Wistar Institute, a National Cancer Institute-designated Cancer Center, sponsor studies. Most studies are done at universities. A few current examples are "mapping genes associated with osteosarcoma in large dog breeds"; a study on canine brain tumors sponsored by the Golden Retriever Foundation; "Characterization of Host and Environmental Risk Factors for Urinary Bladder Cancer in a High Risk Breed (the Scottish Terrier)"; and a study of canine mammary tumors, active at the University of Montreal.[55]

If you have a purebred dog with cancer, he/she may be eligible for a study. "Usually, any dog can participate, but there are always caveats (in regard to previous treatment, etc.). Every study has specifics, so I would recommend contacting me to participate," writes Erika Werne, Grants Director for the AKC Canine Health Foundation.[56] You can reach her at (888) 682-9696.

Over the past decade, researchers have been working vigorously on creating the canine genome. According to Heidi Parker, Ph.D., of the Cancer Genetics Branch, the FHCRC (Fred Hutchinson Cancer Research Center) Canine Genome Project is now rightly labeled the NHGRI Canine Genome Project, part of the Cancer Genetics Branch of the National Human Genome Research Institute in the National Institutes of Health, and the research team resides in Bethesda, Maryland. "We are still intent on identifying the genetic component of cancer susceptibility in dogs. We expect the tremendous increase in resources available to us at NIH to improve our chances of success," writes Parker.[57] Their work includes these projects: Frode Lingaas and Kenine Comstock are studying the mutation that causes a rare form of kidney cancer in German Shepherds; the population structure of dog breeds and "determining how breed relationships can help us find mutations that are shared in multiple breeds from common founders;" studies of malignant histiocytosis (MH is a rare, invariably fatal disorder in which histiocytes, a type of white blood cell, multiply rapidly and invade a wide variety of tissues in a small number of dogs) and lymphoma, performed at universities in the United States and in France.

"We are now in a position to move away from developing the genetic tools and maps necessary to begin a project and can now concentrate our efforts on putting those tools to use in studies of complex disease and disorders," she wrote in October 2004.[58] The completed sequence of the dog genome and a written manuscript outlining the project are due out spring 2005. For more information go to www.genome.gov/11008069.

With an accurate map of genetically transferred diseases available, tests can be developed that would allow carriers to be identified. Then the mating of two carriers, which would produce a dog with a disorder, could be avoided. Surveying the sequence of dogs' genes also will help researchers and doctors better understand human diseases.

CARING FOR OUR BEST FRIENDS

Many dogs are living longer because of new treatments and the use of alternative protocols, better food, and individual care. Here's a heartwarming story, memorialized for posterity for her breed, Norwegian elkhounds, about a dog who survived mast cell tumors. She lives with Sarah Ercolani of Howell, Michigan.

When Daisy was two and a half, her humans found two lumps on her skin. Sometimes these lumps are hard to find on such thick-coated dogs. They went to their veterinarian, Debbie Thayer, D.V.M., at Veterinary Medical Center, in Howell. The veterinarian performed an aspirate test on her bumps to check for cancer. Although she was not sure, she recommended testing and tests came back as possibly cancerous. "Dr. Thayer recommended surgically removing the bumps," writes Daisy in "Daisy's Message." "The lab results told us that I have Mast Cell Tumors, a form of skin cancer in dogs. . . . They took pictures of my insides, samples of my blood, and they told us all about Mast Cell Tumors. My vet had removed extra skin around the tumors called the margins, and the tests showed she successfully removed all the cancer from the area of the tumors." Daisy's tumors were graded as Level II cancer tumors, in the low range.

Although they might come back at any time, X-rays showed that the cancer had not spread. Daisy pleads in a brochure about cancer in dogs, "I want to ask all of you to be sure to check the skin on your dogs for lumps and bumps because you never know. . . . Norwegian Elkhounds . . . and many other breeds of dogs have big, fluffy double coats of hair, making it more difficult to feel bumps, so be sure to give a GOOD feel all over to your beloved doggies frequently so you can detect any growths."[59] Daisy is four now, and since April 2003, when she had her one surgery, the tumors have not reappeared.[60]

On the home front, we continue to love our best friends, and many of us are now feeding our dogs healthier food and exercising them more frequently. Canine agility classes are popular. More no-kill shelters exist; lots of public relations campaigns are waged to inform about spaying and neutering; healthier pet foods and supplements for dogs are more widely available; and an escalating number of books, articles, and Web sites on dog health exist. More animal guardians are seeking out alternative medical methods in addition to the more traditional ones to improve their dogs' lives. Dog parks are becoming more common in many U.S. urban areas, doggie day care helps many people and alleviates some separation anxiety for their pooches, and pooper-scoopers are more widely used—good news for everyone's health.

Domestic dogs need us, and we need dogs, especially considering how many of our lives have become fractured and hectic. We simply must learn how best to care for our best friends.

3 Cats

Cats have been adored, even worshipped, by humans since ancient Egyptian times, approximately four thousand years ago. They were domesticated much later than dogs. Cats beguile us with their beauty, their playfulness and humor, their intelligence, their apparently carefree attitude, and their lack of clinginess. They are quite the opposite in temperament from dogs, and many of us could not conceive of living without them. Cats have become more popular than dogs as domestic companions in the United States, in part because they need a bit less care. They also live longer, and statistically they suffer a slightly lower rate of cancers than dogs.

Currently, approximately 450 million cats live on this planet, the majority of whom are house pets. Every place that is inhabited by humans is also inhabited by cats.[1] The Pet Food Institute estimated that in 1999 there were 74 million cats living in U.S. households; 35 million U.S. households have cats, thus making an average of 2.13 cats per household.[2] The Humane Society of the United States has listed slightly different statistics, based on a 1998 National Pet Owners survey: Three out of ten (or 32 million) U.S. households include at least one cat. Approximately half of those households have one cat; the rest have two or more felines in residence. Cat owners live with more cats in the South (3.2 per household) than in any other region.[3] However, there are also perhaps 60 million feral cats in the United States, often living in colonies and depending on handout meals, products of unwanted pregnancies and abandoned queens.

The Cat Cabana Library, a fairly thorough Web site dedicated to felines, lists forty-two breeds of cats known today, but only thirty-three of them are recognized by the Cat Fanciers' Association, the world's largest registry of pedigreed felines. *Cat Facts* lists about a hundred breeds, falling into five major categories: Persians, other longhairs, British shorthairs, American shorthairs, and Oriental shorthairs. The book notes these categories are not all-inclusive.[4]

Here are three amazing and amusing statistics about cats from the British Cats Protection League. Fewer cat guardians take their animals to the veterinarian than dog guardians: 81.8 percent of cat guardians, as compared to 89.1 percent of dog guardians. If a female cat is not spayed, she could be responsible for about twenty thousand descendants in five years' time. And the oldest cat on record was supposedly a tabby owned by Mrs. Holway of Clayhidon, Devon. Puss lived to be thirty-six and died the day after his birthday, in 1939.[5] Another cat claims this feat, as well. Spike of Bridport, Dorset, England, was a yellow and white cat who died at 31 in 2001. The headline in the BBC News read "World's Oldest Cat Dies." Many cats, however, live into their late teens or early twenties.[6]

SPAYING AND NEUTERING

According to most veterinarians, spaying and neutering cats is a sound idea for at least two reasons. First, it eliminates or helps slow the incredible number of unwanted cat litters around the world. In seven years' time, one female cat and her youngsters can produce 420,000 kittens![7] In just one community, for instance—Key West, Florida—live dozens if not hundreds of feral and semiferal stray cats that, without the help of kind organizations such as Lower Keys Friends of Animals, would not even have enough food to survive. Volunteers trap these animals, have them neutered or spayed at a clinic, and then release them into their original streets or mangroves, where they will no longer be able to reproduce.

But the other reason to spay or neuter is that these procedures can cut down the risk of cancer in both dogs and cats. Spaying a female eliminates the possibility of uterine or ovarian cancer and drastically reduces the risk of breast cancer, particularly if the pet is spayed before her first estrous cycle (the cat's entire reproductive cycle). Cats go into heat at around the age of five to six months. Neutering a male eliminates the possibility of testicular cancer.[8] Disease of the prostate, while avoided in dogs somewhat by neutering, is actually quite rare in cats.

CANCERS

Cats suffer from many varieties of cancer. Indeed, as I noted in chapter 1, the leading nonaccidental cause of death in cats is cancer, at 32 percent. Some of the most frequent types include mammary tumors, fibrosarcomas, mast cell tumors, abdominal masses, lymphosarcomas, thyroid tumors, and vaccine-related feline sarcomas. Feline leukemia, which often leads to other cancers, is the most common infectious disease of cats, affecting 3 percent of cats in the United States.

A cats-only hospital in Charlotte, Vermont, Affectionately Cats, sees approximately twenty-five hundred patients a year. The number of cancer patients has remained steady over the past few years, Denise Kessler, D.V.M., has told me. The most common cancers she sees are lymphosarcomas, primarily in older cats, and fibrosarcomas. Recently, she performed a radical mastectomy on a male cat of seventeen, quite unusual. In the past four and a half years Dr. Kessler has seen three cases of vaccine-induced sarcomas.[9]

Mammary tumors are currently the third most common cancer in felines. Almost 90 percent of them are malignant; the average age of the cat affected is between ten and eleven years old, although our tiger cat, Misty, acquired hers at about age sixteen. These tumors generally metastasize quickly. Many veterinarians believe surgical excision as early as possible is the most effective treatment for any mammary tumor, but read chapter 15 for information on acupuncture and Dr. Are Thoresen's success with using this technique to treat breast cancer in animals. The postsurgical treatment of choice is often chemotherapy, immunotherapy, or radiation.

Veterinarians at the University of Pennsylvania Cancer Center do not recommend taking biopsies of feline mammary tumors for three reasons: Tumors that are at first benign may later become malignant; because each tumor may be a different subtype of mammary tumor, multiple tumors require multiple biopsies (which is potentially dangerous and, to some veterinarians, invasive); and within the same mass of tissue, both benign and malignant tissue may be present. They recommend a surgical procedure to excise all affected or possibly affected tissue as the best course.[10]

Ironically, some of the drugs used commonly for humans are also prescribed for cats. Prednisone, related to cortisone and cortisol, is an immunosuppressive (at high dosages) and is used as part of chemotherapy treatment for such cancers as lymphoma and mast cell tumors. It can also stimulate appetite.[11]

Fibrosarcomas are aggressive and quite difficult to treat. The current estimate is that about one in three thousand cats will develop this cancer; the fibrosarcoma is quite likely to occur at a vaccination site, especially in the neck (see chapter 8, Vaccinations). This is what happened to our sweet eight-year-old calico cat, Puck, in 1997. Although she had two surgeries, our veterinarian's expertise and our own care were unable to lengthen her life appreciably. This was the first case our veterinarian in northern Vermont had seen.

Mike Richards, D.V.M., has written that about 50 percent of the time surgical removal prevents recurrence of fibrosarcomas. He has also recommended radiation therapy when it is economically feasible.[12]

In cats mast cell tumors can be either malignant or benign, and according to Dr. Richards, they are often solitary. He feels that in most cases removing the tumor is sufficient.[13] In a study of cutaneous mast cell tumors in cats at the College of Veterinary Medicine at Washington State University, the one-, two-, and three-year tumor recurrence rates after surgical excision were 16 percent, 19 percent, and 13 percent, respectively. The researchers found that incomplete excision of the tumor did not necessarily correspond with a higher rate of tumor recurrence.[14]

FELINE LEUKEMIA

Feline leukemia (FeLV) is the most common infectious disease of cats, occurring in approximately 3 percent of cats in the United States. It kills more cats than anything except accidents. Discovered in 1964, it is transmitted over time through close contact and constant exposure to an infected cat. It is most commonly transmitted through body secretions, including saliva and urine, over time. Donna Raditic, D.V.M., does not consider it easily passed from cat to cat.[15] A cat infected with FeLV can also have other diseases, including cancerous tumors, leukemia, anemia, and kidney diseases. The most common secondary disease that a cat might develop from FeLV is a cancerous disorder such as lymphoma.

But not all cats who contract the virus develop leukemia. Especially in younger cats, approximately 40 percent have immune systems that neutralize the virus. About 30 percent of the cats with the virus cannot fight it at all, develop other FeLV ailments, and die or are euthanized within three years. Indoor cats with no exposure to other cats are unlikely to develop this or other related diseases. There is no real treatment or cure.[16]

Signs that a cat might have feline leukemia include anemia or lack of pink or red color in the gums, weight loss, a recurring illness, increasing weakness, lethargy, fever, diarrhea, difficulty with breathing, and a yellow color in the mouth and/or the whites of the eyes.[17] In *The New Natural Cat* Anita Frazier adds these symptoms: "depression, repeated persistent infections, failure of wounds to heal . . . tumors revealed by palpation or x-ray . . . and fluid accumulation in chest or abdomen."[18]

A vaccine against FeLV has existed since 1986; this controversial vaccine is discussed more thoroughly in chapter 8. As Alan Spier, a doctor of veterinary medicine at Kansas State University, has said, "There have been some secondary problems associated with the vaccine. Tumors have been reported at the site of injection, though the incidence is rare."[19] Still, this was what happened to our cat Puck.

Lymphosarcoma is the most common cancer associated with feline leukemia. The cancer cells spread throughout the entire body by way of the lymph system. Called the Great Imitator, this disease can mimic other cancers and even other diseases. It can affect all body organs including skin, liver, spleen, intestines, and more. While it can be controlled temporarily with chemotherapy, this is expensive, and remissions may be short. One guardian found a tumor behind her cat's eye, which then invaded through her hard palate, forming a mass on her mouth that made eating nearly impossible. Chemotherapy gave the cat four months; then the tumor returned.[20]

FELINE GENETICS AND CANCER RESEARCH

According to Richard Pitcairn, D.V.M., breeding to meet demand can be extremely dangerous for all animals. For example, during the 1920s Siamese cats became so popular that many were bred to siblings and to parents to produce more kittens. These kittens so weakened the breed that it almost died out. Many pet breeders accept the statistic that between 10 and 25 percent of their litters may be born defective—due in large part to common breeding practices. Dr. Pitcairn notes that Siamese are still more susceptible to disease than other breeds. They suffer "nasal obstruction, chin malformation, cleft palate; retinal degeneration; and weak legs."[21] He adds that among the most common feline problems is cancer of the ear in white-haired cats. They acquire this disease so often because their sensitive ears are especially susceptible to repeated sunburn.[22]

The Morris Animal Foundation, whose work with dogs was detailed in chapter 2, is currently conducting two cat studies. One deals with oral squamous cell carcinoma, cancer of the oral cavity, which often occurs in middle to old age in cats. The other concerns feline lymphocytic plasmacytic enteritis (LPE), a cancer of the gastrointestinal tract with unknown causes.[23]

Another organization deals solely with cats' health issues. The Winn Feline Foundation, founded by the Cat Fanciers' Association in 1968, is headquartered in Manasquan, New Jersey. Since its inception, it has provided nearly $1.5 million dollars for scientific studies to veterinarians. The best news it that "One hundred percent of every donation received by the foundation is used to directly benefit cats. No portion of any donation is used for administrative costs or other expenses."[24]

Since 2000, the foundation has funded several studies related to cancer: one on soft tissue sarcomas at Cornell University; one on oral squamous cell carcinoma at the University of Missouri-Columbia; one on feline mammary gland adenocarcinoma at the University of Illinois; one on feline soft-tissue sarcomas at Colorado State University; one on feline gastrointestinal lymphoma, also at Cornell; one on vaccine-associated sarcomas at the University of Pennsylvania; another on vaccine-associated sarcomas at the University of Wisconsin-Madison; and another at Cornell on feline oral squamous cell carcinoma.[25] According to Susan Little,

D.V.M., vice president of the foundation, few of the studies use client-owned cats, but finding those felines is up to the researcher.[26]

HOMEOPATHY SUCCESS STORY

Finally, here's a happy story about a cat who has recovered from liver cancer, or who is certainly in remission, thanks to some alternative medicine practices administered by Dale Moss, a homeopath in Massachusetts. He wrote this story for my consideration:

> Max, the cat, presented last year at the age of 17. For years she'd been treated by a homeopathic vet for chronic bladder problems and gallbladder duct inflammation, then last year she had a crisis that looked like acute poisoning with lots of thin, clear vomit. She was never right after that: she stopped eating, no longer wanted to be held, and her owner had the impression the cat was leaving her body. The vet treated her with homeopathic *Phosphorus* on the presumption she had cancer; that it was liver cancer was "diagnosed" via an animal communicator. Her owner felt that Max was declining and originally hoped I could simply make her passing more comfortable.
>
> Initially I was reluctant to take the case because there was no proper diagnosis. However, Max had a very clear symptom: she liked to have her abdomen massaged and was better from fairly hard pressure on it. This is what homeopaths would call "strange, rare, and peculiar" in a creature with liver cancer, which presumably would cause the abdomen to be tender to the touch. It's also a symptom of the remedy *Chelidonium*, which is a major remedy for liver problems in general and liver cancer in particular. In other words, the fact that Max was showing signs of needing *Chelidonium* [a homeopathic remedy derived from a plant, a major liver remedy] in my mind confirmed her somewhat unorthodox diagnosis.
>
> It also was a major help that her owner was extraordinarily sensitive to every change in Max's moods and energy.
>
> I put Max on a regimen of *Chelidonium* alternating weekly with a cancer nosode. Both remedies were plussed, as in Ulysses' [Dale's own dog] treatment. At first Max refused to take the remedy, and her owner didn't know how to deal with this. Max, she felt, was

being bossy and trying to be in charge. . . . The trick was to "negotiate" with the cat and persuade her that the owner was merely trying to comply with the cat's desire for help in the best possible way. After doing this, the owner was pleased to report that Max was cooperating fully. In fact, Max eventually got to the point of jumping on her owner's lap each day and staying there through the duration of the treatment.

Max was started at 200c potency last October. There were ups and downs, with symptomatic treatments for constipation and vomiting along the way and an increase to 1M potency in February. Max seemed to be exhausting the remedies' action quickly, which is not a good sign. By May she was still losing weight and wheezing; her eyes were also running more. Worse, she was favoring her belly, which suggested that *Chelidonium* might no longer be the correct remedy.

Instead of changing remedies, however, I upped the potency to 10M. By July she was throwing up once or twice a week and urinating on the floor. The animal communicator told the owner that the cancer had metastasized and was now throughout Max's body. Her owner reported that Max seemed unhappy and tired, but her fur, which the owner used as a gauge to the cat's health, continued to be fluffy and gray. She was noticeably suffering from the hot weather, so I treated her for that with another liver support remedy in addition to continuing with the plussing regimen. [Plussing means dissolving a high-potency remedy in distilled water, taking 10 doses by dropper or teaspoon a day, usually one dose every 15 minutes, over the timeframe of two and a half hours.]

By September, however, the situation had turned around. Max was more energetic, more affectionate, and outgoing. Friends couldn't believe this was the same cat—her personality had changed so! Even better news came when the animal communicator told us that the higher potency had boosted Max's vital force enough to kill off the metastases and that the original tumor was shrinking.

Max still [in September 2004] has some minor health issues, mainly because of her age and the fact that her energy is still going into fighting off the cancer. But she seems well on the way to being cured.[27]

4 Other Small Animals

FERRETS

In the past dozen or so years ferrets have become exceedingly popular as pocket pets. However, they are not new as animal companions. Ferrets have served as companions to humans since around 1200 B.C. Aristotle reportedly mentioned the ferret in his works.[1]

Unfortunately, in large part because of overbreeding to meet the current demand, ferrets now suffer from several different cancers. As I noted in chapter 1, an October 1997 Morris Animal Foundation study identified cancer as the primary cause of disease-related deaths among these small animals, at 33 percent.[2]

Ferrets can be fascinating and entertaining companions, and are especially suited to apartment living. They can be litter-box trained but also need a cage because they are incredibly active and must be restricted when you are not around. They may live for eight to twelve years and require annual vaccines, neutering, and descenting because they have a somewhat wild odor. In addition, they can catch colds and flu easily from humans.[3] Some are aggressive, but most are merely mischievous; they love to have fun. Be aware, though, that it is illegal to keep them as pets in some parts of the United States.

The Humane Society of the United States cautions people to be serious if they want to live with ferrets: "Ferrets are very different from more traditional companion animals such as dogs and cats. They are marketed by the pet industry as 'unusual,' but individuals considering adopting a ferret should be wary of the industry's claims that unusual pets are easy to care for. Ferrets require a high level of commitment to be cared for responsibly and humanely." They also recommend that small children "never be left unsupervised with ferrets (or with any other companion animals)."[4]

Care

Several things need to be done to make sure your ferret stays well. Here are a few suggestions from Alicia Drakiotes, education coordinator for Ferret Wise, a Web page of Petsville Library:

+ Keep track of your animal's weight.
+ Check her coat, which should be shiny and glossy, except during seasonal changes.
+ Make sure her coat is not dry or flaky.
+ Her eyes should be clear and bright with no discharge.
+ Keep her ears clean—they should be pink and have no smell.
+ The ferret's gums should be pink, not pale.
+ Check her entire body for any lumps or bumps, just as you would check any animal companion.
+ Her feet and pads should not dry out or crack.
+ The genitalia should have no swelling or signs of irritation.
+ And finally, if your ferret coughs or gasps often, check with your vet.[5]

Cancers

Several cancers do exist in these two- to three-pound animals. In *Ferrets, Rabbits, and Rodents: Clinical Medicine and Surgery,* author Susan A. Brown, D.V.M., writes, "The probability is excellent that a ferret in the United States will develop one or more neoplastic (cancerous) diseases by the time it reaches five years of age." She adds, "In no other country where ferrets are kept as pets has such an overwhelming incidence of cancer in ferrets been reported."[6]

Dr. Brown lists the following as possible causes of the rise in cancer, although she states there is no consensus on them:

+ Genetic predisposition, perhaps caused by large ferret-breeding facilities, which might inadvertently "recycle" genetic factors that result in cancers.

+ Early neutering of ferrets at five to six weeks of age—a common practice within the U.S. pet industry for preventing other diseases and for making animals more marketable.

+ Lack of natural photoperiod or exposure to natural sunlight. Ferrets are extremely sensitive to light. In the United States most ferrets are housed indoors. In Europe and Australia the majority of ferrets kept as companions are housed outdoors all year.

+ Diet. In the United States ferrets are fed mostly processed dry cat food or ferret food. Brown believes that although the quality of such food is better than it was in the past, diet may still play a part in causing cancers. In Europe and Australia many ferret owners feed their small companions a more natural diet: rabbits, mice, and rats.

+ Infectious agents. In the case of lymphoma, some studies also point to a viral cause.[7]

Kevin Fitzgerald, D.V.M., has said that he sees more and more cancer in ferrets because of too much inbreeding on ferret farms. He also points out that anesthesia is a problem; if they need surgery, these animals can easily die because their small size makes appropriate anesthesia levels extremely difficult to determine.[8]

Two types of cancer seem to occur quite regularly in ferrets. The first is insulinoma, which often occurs at three years of age or older. These small tumors of the beta cells in the pancreas secrete extra insulin. A ferret with this disease becomes hypoglycemic—it does not have enough sugar to function properly. According to Alicia Drakiotes, warning signs of this disease include being less playful; becoming weak and showing signs of muscle weakness, especially in the hind end; possibly some bobbing of the head; excessive salivation and pawing at the mouth; weight loss and dull coat; and, the worst, seizures. During a seizure the animal may become unresponsive to outside stimulation. If this happens to your ferret, advises Drakiotes, you must give her something sugary immediately to raise her blood sugar level. Corn syrup, honey, or maple syrup applied to the ferret's gums with a cotton swab is appropriate, after which you should contact a veterinarian immediately. Drakiotes recommends calling the veterinarian if you note any of these warning signs.[9]

Early detection with this disease, as with all cancers, is one way to permit your animal to successfully battle the illness and live longer. In *An Owner's Guide to a Happy Healthy Pet: The Ferret,* author Mary R. Shefferman says that initial lethargy is the most common symptom of insulinoma, usually occurring at three to four years, and is often misinterpreted as simply part of aging. She stresses the importance of early detection as well.[10]

According to Drakiotes's article "Insulinoma in Ferrets," two treatments exist for insulinoma. The first is surgery—removing the tumors on the pancreas. However, there has been a high rate of recurrence, averaging fourteen to sixteen months after surgery. The second choice is medication. Two oral drugs exist. One is Prednisolone (or Pedia-Pred, a liquid children's version). This stimulates the liver to produce more glucose, or sugar, and is fairly inexpensive, though it can cause liver damage and other problems if given over a period of time. The other medication is Proglycem of Diazoxide, which inhibits insulin secretion. This is expensive; a one-ounce bottle costs more than $100 and may last only a month. Some ferret owners use both drugs, but Drakiotes recommends surgery as the best route for gaining more time and a better quality of life for your ferret.[11]

The second type of cancer that affects ferrets of all ages, equally in both sexes, is lymphosarcoma (which is, of course, also common in dogs and cats). This may occur in many organs of the body; it may be found in bone marrow, lymph nodes, liver, spleen, intestines, and spinal cord. It is often widespread, occurring in many sites. According to Ruth Adams, D.V.M., of the Ferret Clinic, lymphosarcoma may be caused by a virus (somewhat akin to the feline leukemia virus in cats), though this possibility has not yet been fully substantiated. Symptoms of this disease may include lethargy, coughing, fever, and difficulty with breathing. Chronic weight loss is one of the most common. A veterinarian may find enlarged peripheral lymph nodes or an enlarged spleen. There also may be masses in the abdomen or chest.[12] Ultrasound is frequently used to diagnostically differentiate between a lymphoma and cardiac disease.[13]

For lymphosarcoma, Dr. Adams recommends chemotherapy. The initial improvement with some forms can be dramatic, but the ferret's progress must be followed with serial blood tests to make sure the treatment is not greatly damaging the bone marrow's blood-producing cells. Ferrets tolerate chemotherapy quite well, with few side effects. However, while remissions of six to twelve months are possible, this disease is rarely cured.[14]

Another type of cancer frequently seen in ferrets—indeed, the most common of liver ailments in these small creatures—is hepatic neoplasia. Writer Thomas J. Burke states that tumors of the skin and subcutis are also found and are frequently malignant. He notes a few additional commonly reported cancers, including squamous cell carcinomas, mast cell tumors, and adenocarcinomas of sebaceous and perianal glands.[15]

As for treatments, herbal therapies are beginning to be used for ferrets, as explained by Dian Bodofsky in her Web article, "Herbal Therapy . . . Hope for Our Ferrets." She is using herbs with the full cooperation of her veterinarian; they are both monitoring the results. She uses Alfalfa Leaf 1,2 for anemia and balancing the hormones when treating hypo- and hyperestrogenism; Hawthorne Supreme 1,2 for heart conditions; and Pau d'Arco 1,2 for its anticancer properties and usefulness in chronic health imbalances. Her eight-year-old ferret Butter was diagnosed with lymphoma in November 1994 and in 1998 was still in remission after receiving chemotherapy. He was started on Pau d'Arco in May 1997, receiving five drops twice a day mixed with fifty milligrams of vitamin C, one teaspoon of Hill's a/d (a prescription pet food available through veterinarians), and one teaspoon of water. Butter showed an increase in energy and appetite in a few days and also showed a slight increase in fur growth. Even though she had relatively speedy results, Bodofsky warns that changes with herbs can be gradual. She advises animal guardians to remain patient.[16]

GUINEA PIGS

Another popular pocket pet—especially with small children—is the guinea pig, or cavy. These animal companions are relatively easy to care for and are very small. They generally live to be between five and eight years old.

Care

Guinea pigs should eat a balanced diet of hay, pellets, and fresh fruits and vegetables. The latter are especially important because guinea pigs cannot manufacture their own vitamin C. Pellets contain vitamin C, but most experts believe it is important to supplement them. Other C sources include red and green bell peppers, broccoli, kale, cabbage, spinach, chicory, and leaf lettuces. Ceramic dishes are best for feeding, as is true for most animals. Do not feed in plastic, because this can precipitate various conditions, including chin acne.

Symptoms that might warrant immediate attention by a veterinarian include decreased appetite, weight loss or gain, discharge from eyes or nose, diarrhea, limping, lethargy, hair loss, and lumps or bumps.[17]

Cancers

Even guinea pigs develop tumors, which can include often-benign skin and subcutaneous tumors. Sows, middle-aged to older females, can develop ovarian cysts as early as fifteen months, though they most frequently occur in females three or more years old. These cysts tend to be filled with fluid, and if one bursts it can likely lead to death.

Some of these tumors may be as large as two and a half inches in diameter, astonishing if you think of the size of the creature, but they rarely metastasize. One obvious sign of this type of growth is when both sides of the body start balding, just forward of the hips. Other signs of these growths include depression, weakness, or collapse from a spontaneous intra-abdominal hemorrhage. An ovariohysterectomy is a possible solution, if it is done at the right time. This process is similar to that performed on ferrets, dogs, and cats.[18] The veterinarians on the Cavy Care Web site recommend spaying to remove the ovaries and the uterus to prevent these cancers.[19]

RABBITS

The domestic rabbit is one more popular home companion susceptible to some forms of cancer. Because rabbits are small and fuzzy, and look so silky and adorable, people often buy them on a whim with little knowledge of their needs. We do not instinctively know as much about rabbits as we do about dogs and cats, because most of us have never lived with them. In fact, rabbits are quite fussy about their food and their homes and can be fragile and frail and ornery. They are sometimes nervous and scare easily—and generally do not like to be too close to children, who can squeeze too hard. However, rabbits are affectionate, intelligent, and amusing animals, and can make delightful companions who give a lot of love and laughter. In the best of situations they may live eight to ten years.

More than fifty breeds of rabbits have been domesticated since the Middle Ages. They have long been popular as animal companions in the United Kingdom and now are quite popular in the United States as well.

A friend and colleague, Rebecca Werner of Huntington, Vermont, who has always lived with rabbits, describes their particular appeal, "Rabbits lend uncommon sensitivity and quietness to an often uncivil and unkind world. When you have a high stress job, they can help bring balance into your life—they allow you to think in silence."[20]

Care

To keep a rabbit happy and healthy, you should keep her on a regular feeding schedule of good food. High-quality rabbit pellets, fresh vegetables and fruits, and alfalfa hay are the main ingredients in such a diet. Sometimes you can add rabbit vitamins as a supplement. Keep your animal's water fresh and pure, too. If you use regular tap water, rinse the dishes daily, and wash and disinfect them weekly. If you use a piped-water system, check the valves daily and flush the entire system on a regular basis.

Rabbits also require some hands-on care. They need regular grooming, especially when they are shedding; like cats, they develop hairballs, and because they do not vomit, they ingest these. In addition to regular brushing they appreciate some playtime each day. According to rabbit care advice administered by the Humane Society of the United States, "because rabbits groom each other around the eyes, ears, top of the nose, top of the head, and down the back, they'll think of you as a kindred spirit if you pat them there, too."[21]

A rabbit's cage must be cleaned daily, which includes cleaning or changing some form of litter or bedding. This bedding should be non-toxic and absorbent. Clumping cat litters have been known to cause internal blockages, cancer, and respiratory disease. Some rabbits ingest litter and dislike dusty kinds. Good choices are sand, recycled paper-based litter, hay, straw, dried grass, and corncob litter. Using a litter box with wire covering the drop pan is recommended.[22] The Humane Society of the United States recommends organic litters made of oats, paper, alfalfa, or citrus. Hay is an option but requires more frequent changing because rabbits like to eat it.[23]

Since the mid-1970s a heated debate has raged about the use of certain rabbit litters, especially softwood litters such as pine shavings or cedar chips. They have been found to cause liver disease and respiratory problems in small animals. According to Carolina James of the Rabbit Charity, a nonprofit rescue and education group in the United Kingdom, the problem is the natural volatile chemicals, or phenols, in the wood. These are caustic, poisonous, acidic compounds routinely diluted for use in disinfectants. At high levels of contact, you risk damage to the liver and kidneys. At lower levels, however, the damage to the liver may not be fatal, but it will depress the immune system. This can leave the rabbit vulnerable to infections, especially of the respiratory tract. If you choose to use a softwood bedding, it is generally best to keep it in a large, open, well-ventilated area. Be aware that the dust in the sawdust and shavings can irritate rabbits' eyes.[24] Also see chapter 5 for more information on litters.

A healthy rabbit has a coat that is shiny and pliable and springs back immediately after you touch it. When an animal is stressed, either physically or emotionally, her immune system becomes weakened, which gives bacteria a chance to establish. Signs that a rabbit may have a bacterial infection include a runny nose or eyes, labored breathing, lack of coordination, paralysis of limbs, incontinence, a fever higher than the normal 102°F, inflammation or swelling, pus, and loss of appetite. Many rabbits develop abscesses in the middle ear, lymph nodes, eyes, or skin, which are sometimes treated with drugs such as tetracycline in the drinking water.[25]

Cancers

Although less is known about the incidence of cancer in rabbits than in cats and dogs, the disease does exist. In fact, one veterinarian in the Burlington, Vermont, area told me that rabbits can get any cancer that humans can! And as I noted in chapter 1, cancer is the leading cause of disease-related death among rabbits, at 28 percent.

The variety of cancer that occurs most regularly is uterine cancer (adenocarcinoma), usually in unspayed rabbits over the age of two. The British Houserabbit Association lists the risk of fatal reproductive cancer for an unspayed female rabbit at approximately 85 percent, especially as she ages.[26] A U.S. source, Joanne Paul-Murphy, D.V.M., says that 50 to 80 percent of rabbits older than four years (especially certain breeds—tan, French silver, Havana, and Dutch) have a chance of acquiring this disease.[27] Yet another source, Cinnamon Gimness, manager of The Bunny House at Best Friends Animal Society, says that studies indicate that: "up to eighty percent of unspayed female rabbits will get uterine and/or ovarian cancer between two and five years of age," and that a high percentage of male rabbits will develop testicular cancer if not neutered.[28]

A doe at risk for uterine cancer typically has a history of reproductive disturbance in the six to ten months before the tumor became obvious to the touch. Typical problems might be a small litter size, stillborns, or the mother deserting her litter. While the tumors are developing (they are slow to develop), other problems might arise: difficulty kindling, litter retention in utero, abdominal pregnancy, and fetal resorption are more likely than usual. The tumors are usually multiple; their growth rates vary. The time from detection to death from metastases ranges from one to two years.[29]

The classic study of this rabbit cancer was completed in 1958 by H. S. N. Greene. It showed that 4 percent of does had uterine cancer at two to three years of age; the number rose to 80 percent at five or six years of age. Another study in 1962 found that the breed did not seem to make a difference in these statistics; nor did whether or not the rabbit had been bred.[30]

Uterine cancer can spread to other organs such as the liver, the lungs, and even the skin; it is not treatable once it reaches this point.[31] Complications such as mastitis, pregnancy toxemia, and other conditions are common. The doe can easily die.

However, according to the British Houserabbit Association's authors Linda Dykes and Owen Davies, an important early sign to watch for is occasional blood in the urine. Rabbits with early tumors may be saved if they are spayed when the cancer is still entirely within the uterus, before it has begun to metastasize. According to Dr. Paul-Murphy, if the tumor is contained within the uterus, the prognosis is good with an ovariohysterectomy. If local invasion of tumors is still observed, it is important to reexamine the rabbit every six months for one to two years after the surgery. Paul-Murphy notes that successful chemotherapy for this type of tumor has not yet been reported.[32]

Another type of cancer occasionally found in female rabbits is breast cancer. Although not common, when it does occur it spreads rapidly and is difficult to treat. Spaying before age two helps prevent this disease. The most common form of mammary cancer is malignant, and it is almost always associated with uterine cancer.

In males, testicular cancer does occur but is uncommon. Abscesses, often from bite wounds from other rabbits, and hematomas (blood-filled areas) are more common.[33]

Spaying and Neutering

All rabbit experts recommend spaying and neutering of rabbits if you are not breeding them. If you buy a rabbit and are not sure whether she has been altered, take her to the vet. Aside from averting possible disease, spaying and neutering also reduce infections due to bites and scratches, and reduce susceptibility to urinary infections in general.[34] Rabbits who are neutered tend to be less aggressive and territorial. Neutered male rabbits stop spraying urine (even if they are older when neutered).[35]

But there are a few cautions. Spaying rabbits, which involves removal of the uterus and both ovaries, is somewhat risky. Castration of the males removes the testicles via an incision in the scrotum or the lower abdomen and is a much more straightforward procedure. In the past some anesthesias have been extremely dangerous—even lethal—to rabbits, especially does. Fortunately, they have improved of late.[36] However, individual rabbits have varying sensitivity to the depressant effects of anesthesia. There is a narrow range between the necessary amount of anesthetic and a toxic dose; mortality following anesthesia and surgery is not uncommon in rabbits. A short anesthetic time is generally recommended, and clinicians need to watch closely for individual responses to the drugs. Both injectable and inhalant anesthesias may be used effectively.[37]

When a vet anesthetizes your rabbit, be sure he or she has done this surgery on a rabbit before. Not all surgical products that are used on cats and dogs can be used on bunnies. Neutering can be done at four to six months; for the doe, spaying can be done at six months. With giant breeds, sometimes surgery is postponed to the ninth month. Overall, the safest time for surgery is four months to one year, although some five- and six-year-old rabbits can withstand it. For rabbits more than one year old, a basic preoperative blood panel is recommended, which checks for anemia, high liver enzymes, and kidney function. If the blood test looks good, surgery will probably be safe. If not, you can postpone surgery.

The House Rabbit Society recommends not putting your rabbit on a fast before surgery; recovery is quicker if the animal does not miss a meal. Because they do not vomit, rabbits can eat and drink water before surgery. Changes in diet can upset a rabbit's digestive tract and cause problems after surgery in her recovery. If the rabbit is exceptionally high strung, the vet can sedate her with preanesthetic before gas is given. This is especially important when the vet uses halothane as the gas.

After surgery the rabbit is generally confined to a clean, disinfected cage for two days for males, or five to six days for females. The animal's stools may be unusual for a couple of days. If the rabbit likes to sleep in her litter box, remove it: This could contaminate the sutured area. Check the sutures daily to see that they are not becoming swollen and are free of discharge. Males and females should be separated for two weeks, in case of stored sperm and to allow incisions to heal before any sexual activity. Neutered pairs continue to be sexually active. Most rabbits are able to eat immediately following surgery, but some may refuse food for a couple of days.[38] However, if your pet does not eat within forty-eight hours or seems terribly uncomfortable, consult your veterinarian.[39]

For rabbits who are obese or have an illness or disease, the Rabbit Charity does not recommend any surgeries, even routine neutering. The group recommends that the animal first be put on a diet or that any diseases be attended to prior to any major surgery.[40]

5 Environmental Concerns

According to the National Cancer Institute, each type of cancer has its own known or suspected risk factors, and all cancers are almost always caused by a combination of factors that interact in ways "not yet fully understood."[1]

Obviously, some of these factors are environmental, and many come to us and our animal companions through what we ingest—our diet and our drinking water. These two topics will be covered in chapter 6, Drinking Water, and chapter 7, Nutrition. But there are also many other risks involved with daily life that affect and may cause disease—or even death—in both human and nonhuman animals.

DANGERS IN THE HOUSE

Some of the materials with which you built your residence or furnished it may lead to health problems. In *Earl Mindell's Nutrition and Health for Dogs* (coauthored with Elizabeth Renaghan), Mindell writes at great length about the importance of maintaining a strong immune system, and how pollution in our homes can diminish this possibility. The Environmental Protection Agency (EPA) conducted studies of air pollution levels both indoors and outdoors for five years. They found that indoor pollution levels are one hundred to two hundred times higher. Mindell recommends cleaning all filters, ducts, and vents often, or you and your animals could be breathing asbestos, pollens, pesticides, tobacco, dust mites, mildew, bacteria, and a host of other unhealthy agents.

If you are building or remodeling a home, look for products that say "toxin-free" on the label. Carpets especially are troublesome. Look for a "green label" stating that the product has met voluntary emissions criteria. It is a good idea to have the retailer air out your new carpet, and for you to air out your home once the carpet is installed. Rubber latex in carpet backing and carpet adhesive often emits toxic fumes. This can cause a variety of ailments, including headaches, vomiting, nausea, and irritated eyes. Paints are important to consider, too. Oil- or latex-based paints contain approximately three hundred toxic substances. The fumes often linger and can cause all sorts of ailments for both humans and domestic animals. Try to choose paints labeled "a clean air choice." When you paint, keep your animals outside or even at a friend's house, and leave your windows open.

Mindell recommends against softwood plywood, waferboard, or strand board over pressed woods, many of which contain a toxin called urea formaldehyde. Again, these products can cause nausea along with throat, lung, and skin irritations, and more. "The Environmental Protection Agency estimates that in the United States we spend over one billion dollars on medical costs for cancer and heart disease caused by indoor pollutants," writes Mindell. These indoor pollutants are twice as toxic to a dog (and presumably to a cat or ferret) half the size of an adult, so think of the illness we could help avert by being more careful and environmentally conscious![2]

In my first edition, I omitted radon as I have never had to deal with this issue in our two homes. We have been lucky. According to the EPA, "Radon is the second leading cause of lung cancer. Nearly one in 15 homes in the U.S. has a high level of indoor radon. The U.S. Surgeon General and EPA recommend all homes be tested for radon." The good news is that a house with radon can be "fixed."[3]

The list of what is toxic or dangerous to your animal companions does not end here. Think of things you might consider for children's safety, too—your medications, your cleaning products, your mouse or rat traps. Acetaminophen can do significant tissue damage to an animal; only one extra-strength tablet can kill a cat. Aspirin, ibuprofen, and phenylbutazone are less dangerous but should never be used unless specified by a veterinarian. Naproxen is toxic to cats but can be used for dogs. The ASPCA Animal Poison Control Center advises to immediately throw away any drugs that fall on the floor.[4]

Ant poisons and insecticides contain different active ingredients, generally broken into two categories: organophosphates and carbamates (also in flea products). Both have toxic effects that cause an excess of the neurotransmitter acetylcholine to accumulate in the body. An excess or overdose of this can cause death.

Chocolate is dangerous because theobromine and caffeine, two of its ingredients, are toxic to animals. Of most concern is the true baking-type chocolate. Generally chocolate candies can be tolerated in fair amounts. If you are at all concerned about the danger of the kind or quantity ingested by an animal companion, call your animal care provider. Another sweet that can prove toxic to canines is sugar-free candy or gum, which contains xylitol. Based on 40-plus related cases in 2003 and 2004, the Animal Poison Control Center (APCC) found that dogs "may develop a sudden drop in blood sugar, resulting in depression, loss of coordination and seizures." The signs can develop as quickly as 30 minutes after ingestion; animal guardians should seek veterinary help immediately.[5] Grapes and raisins can also be toxic. Between April 2003 and April 2004, the ASPCA Animal Poison Control Center studied 140 related cases, each of one or more dogs who "ingested varying amounts of raisins or grapes." They do not know yet if all canines are susceptible, stated Dana Farbman, Certified Veterinary Technician (CVT) at the ASPCA.[6]

Even more dangerous is antifreeze (ethylene glycol), which animals sometimes drink from puddles in cold climates such as mine. Half a teaspoon per pound for a dog can be a toxic dose—even less for a cat. The poison affects kidney function, which in turn results in impaired neurological function. It can bring on depression, vomiting, seizures, and loss of coordination.

The next category of dangerous products includes dozens of household cleaning agents such as toilet bowl cleaners, bleaches, and detergents. These can destroy tissue by acid or alkaline burns, by dissolving through tissue membranes, by being absorbed into the bloodstream, and by causing generalized illness and other symptoms. Many of these products contain organic chemicals, which can release organic compounds when used and even, to some extent, when they are stored. According to the U.S. Environmental Protection Agency's Total Exposure Assessment Methodology (TEAM), "studies found levels of about a dozen common organic pollutants to be 2 to 5 times higher inside homes than outside," in both rural and urban settings. Sources to be cautious of are "household products including: paints, paint strippers, and other solvents; wood preservatives; aerosol sprays; cleansers and disinfectants; moth repellents and air fresheners; stored fuels and automotive products; hobby supplies; and dry-cleaned clothing." These may damage the liver, kidney, and central nervous system and "some organics can cause cancer in animals."[7]

In an article titled "Spring Cleaning: Using Pet-Safe Products to Clean Your Home," writer Amy Carlton includes this list of particularly hazardous chemicals often found in commercial cleaning products:

+ Perchloroethylene is a stain remover that is a known animal carcinogen.
+ Amyl acetate is found in furniture polish.
+ Artificial colors and fragrances with no cleaning value can cause allergic reactions or irritations.
+ Benzene is a carcinogen found in many detergents and oven cleaning supplies.
+ Naphthalene, a cousin of benzene linked to skin allergies, cataracts, and kidney problems, is often contained in deodorizers and carpet cleaners.

Carlton recommends chemical-free products by companies such as Seventh Generation, Earth Rite, and Harmony, or making your own cleaning supplies with items such as baking soda, lemon juice, and other inexpensive, safe substitutes for those chemical products.[8]

In addition, flea products—which I will cover at greater length later in this chapter, are not as safe as they seem, especially if they are not used as directed. Some may actually be carcinogenic. If your animal shows any abnormal reaction—scratching, depression, vomiting, diarrhea, excessive salivation—stop using them and contact your animal health care provider.

Lead poisoning is possible if small animals ingest an object containing lead, such as a battery, a toy, or a fishing weight. Pets may also swallow lead-containing paint, caulk, motor oil, or other products. Dogs can contract zinc poisoning if they ingest pennies. This does not happen often, thankfully, but can cause weakness, trembling, and loss of appetite if it does. Keep those pennies in that jar.

Finally, rodenticides—intended to kill rats, mice, and their small cousins—are some of the deadliest substances for other animals. These are most often found in garages or in barns in rural settings. Even if these products are kept in a safe container far from your animal's reach, a dog or cat can easily be poisoned by eating a rodent that has consumed a rodenticide. Dana Farbman of the ASPCA said, "If a pet ingests a rodenticide, potentially serious or even life-threatening problems can result, such as bleeding, seizures, or damage to the kidneys and other vital organs."[9] It is best, then, to simply avoid using them altogether.[10]

OUTDOOR DANGERS

Sun can hurt animals just as it can humans. They, too, develop skin cancers. Excessive exposure to sunlight can especially create risk for areas without hair or pigmentation. In cats these include the pink tip of the nose, the eyelids, and the ear region. For dogs, fair complexions and high exposure on the underbelly or the inside of the back legs can cause problems. Skin cancer often develops in pointers, bull terriers, pit bulls, and Dalmatians in high mountain areas with especially strong ultraviolet light, says Dr. Barbara E. Kitchell, oncologist and veterinarian at the University of Illinois Veterinary Medicine Teaching Hospital at Urbana.[11] Dr. Rodney Page, D.V.M., director of the Comparative Cancer Program at Cornell University's College of Veterinary Medicine, stresses the importance of protecting your dog from direct sunlight, "especially if the animal is lightly pigmented, or unpigmented (pure white). Periodically check your dog's skin, lymph nodes, paws, nails and inside of its mouth and look for any unusual lumps or sores. This should be done every two or three months. It's especially important as the dog grows older."[12]

A hospital-based study of companion dogs examined the risk of exposure to 2,4-dichlorophenoxyacetic acid (2,4-D) herbicides used in lawn care. After examining almost five hundred cases and more than nine hundred tumor and nontumor controls, researchers found a twofold increase in malignant canine lymphomas where lawns had four or more applications a year. The findings are consistent with occupational studies on humans exposed to 2,4-D.[13]

The April 15, 2005 issue of the *Journal of the American Veterinary Medical Association* included an article on herbicide exposure risks to dogs. Lawrence T. Glickman, V.M.D., Dr.PH, of Purdue University and colleagues studied dogs to determine whether exposure was associated with "an increased risk of the most common cancer of the urinary bladder in dogs, transitional cell carcinoma (TCC). The prevalence of TCC in dogs examined at veterinary teaching hospitals in North America increased by more than 600% between 1975 and 1995." The investigators determined that the risk of TCC was "significantly increased" in dogs exposed to "lawns or gardens treated with both herbicides and insecticides or with herbicides alone." At most risk are terriers, particularly Scottish Terriers.[14]

Another cancer possibly resulting from outdoor exposure to herbicides, pesticides, or automobile pollution is nasal sinus cancer. Dogs have a much higher rate of this than do humans, possibly because they happily sniff every inch of the ground more readily than we do.[15]

There are twenty thousand pesticide products on the U.S. Market, which means that we and our children and animals are exposed to them all the time—at home, in office buildings, in schools. The Environmental Protection Agency has announced, "New research indicates that pesticides can cause cancer, reproductive problems and developmental disorders." The EPA and other agencies, such as the Food and Drug Administration and the Agriculture and Justice departments, do monitor the uses of pesticides, but we still need to do our part to protect our families. In at least one study, "Laboratory rodents exposed to such chemicals [as exist in commercial pesticides] suffer from higher rates of certain types of cancer, and become more aggressive and hyperactive," writes David Hosansky in "Regulating Pesticides," for CQ Researcher.[16] Although pesticides may come to us through residues on food, another source is more critical, "The somewhat casual use of pesticides in yards, gardens, parks is a much more important target for pesticide reduction," noted Sheila Zahm, deputy director of the division of cancer epidemiology and genetics at the National Cancer Institute.[17]

Always read labels; a popular product such as TrueGreen Chemlawn, which uses beautiful Dalmatian dogs to advertise on its trucks, contains some carcinogenic active ingredients. Chemlawn (its EPA Registered Name is Acme aqueous pyrenone garden spray) contains piperonyl butoxide, a possible carcinogen, and Pyrethrins, which are highly toxic carcinogens.[18] Each time I see one of its trucks around town, I admire the happy and healthy-looking Dalmation on the side. Then, when I look at the complaints filed against the company and the ingredients of the lawn care product, I feel particularly misled.

The EPA does classify pesticides for their carcinogenicity. As of the newest report in July 19, 2004, they have evaluated hundreds of chemicals. The two categories most worrisome are, obviously, "carcinogenic to humans," which means there is "compelling evidence of carcinogenicity in animals . . ." and "likely to be carcinogenic to humans" where the experimental evidence gathered shows "animal carcinogenicity by a mode or modes of action that are relevant or assumed to be relevant to humans." In other words, these chemicals are tested on rats and mice. In the first category, "Carcinogenic to humans" and, therefore, to animals, are these chemicals: arsenic acid; arsenic pentoxide; arsenate, sodium; benzene; and chromium (VI). But under the second category, those that show "animal carcinogenicity," there are more than one hundred. These range from acetaldehyde to aldrin to azobenzene to captan to chlordane to DDD, DDE, and DDT, and so on. A report "Chemicals Evaluated for Carcinogenic Potential" is available through the EPA.[19]

Many studies have linked a large percentage of feline leukemias to environmental carcinogens. These include chemicals in the air, water, and food; indoor and outdoor cleaners; and insecticides. Flea sprays and collars are suspect, too. (For the possible role of vaccinations in feline leukemia, see chapter 8.)

In *Are You Poisoning Your Pets?* Nina Anderson and Howard Peiper list chlordane, DDT, and lindane (this is categorized as showing "suggestive evidence of carcinogenicity" on the EPA document mentioned above) as a few agricultural sprays that are "potential killers" or that can have long-term effects on the body. A DDT by-product, DDE, has even been found in tumors of some breast cancer patients. "Female pets are at risk, too," these authors note.[20]

According to recent news from Defenders of Wildlife, twenty consumer and environmental groups have asked Home Depot and Lowe's Home Improvement "to protect the health of children, families, pets and the environment and to reconsider the sale of 'weed and feed' due to its hazards and environmental pollution." In Canada, seventy municipalities, including Toronto, Quebec, and Halifax, have either banned or restricted the use of lawn pesticides.[21]

GOLF IS NOT JUST A GAME

Last January I met a retired businessman turned full-time sailor who had recently lost his beloved hunting dog, an Italian spinone *(spinone Italiano),* to lung cancer. The dog was only three and a half years old. His owner attributes the cancer primarily to pesticides and herbicides used on the golf course next door to them in rural Kentucky. The breed is not known for a high rate of cancer.

Golf courses are apparently quite toxic to both humans and animals. A study of causes of death among golf course superintendents indicated a statistically significant number of deaths attributable to non-Hodgkin's lymphoma and brain cancer between 1970 and 1992.[22]

According to a related report by Jared Baragar, chemicals used on golf courses have caused cancer, birth defects, nerve damage, and heart disturbances. Caddies also suffer eye problems, throat and congestion problems, headaches, and more. Baragar notes that a single eighteen-hole golf course can, in one year, use fifty thousand pounds of dry and liquid chemicals. The Global Anti-Golf Movement states that golf courses "destroy natural ecosystems, contaminate the environment, and threaten human health."[23] And clearly animal health as well.

SECONDHAND TOBACCO SMOKE

Tobacco smoke can injure animals just as it injures us. Secondhand smoke causes about three thousand lung cancer deaths a year among humans in the United States. Children of parents who smoke have more respiratory symptoms and more infections, as well as more evidence of reduced lung function, than do those of nonsmoking parents. Cigarettes contain approximately sixty compounds that are either carcinogens, tumor initiators (these can result in irreversible changes in normal cells), or tumor promoters (which may lead to tumor growth once cell changes commence). A few of these substances are tar, carbon monoxide, phenols, ammonia, benzene, and nicotine.[24]

TOYS AND TREATS

Now let's consider the toys you so thoughtfully buy your dog or cat, some of which are actually quite dangerous. At the top of the list for dogs are most rawhide chews. Even though they give pooches a long-lasting treat, keep them amused when you are too busy to take a walk, and can help in reducing dental problems, they have latent dangers as well. Dogs can choke on rawhide ends and can sustain intestinal blockage; if you do give your dogs these toys, you should supervise their happy chewing.

But there are problems with the rawhide material itself. How are these things made? Fresh hides must be preserved, the hair removed, and the hides cured to prevent them from spoiling. Many of the least-expensive chews come from Asia, where uncontrolled chemical usage has caused massive pollution in rivers and aquifers. (According to an investigative article on this topic, one company, IPSD of San Diego, California, sold rawhide products from Argentina, Canada, China, Ecuador, and Thailand, where cheap hides could be had.) Some of the residues found in poorly processed animal hides are lead, arsenic, mercury, chromium salts, and formaldehyde. The U.S. Department of Agriculture (USDA) has jurisdiction over animal products imported into this country but requires only an import license and a certificate of origin. Perhaps U.S. rawhides are safer, but chemical processing happens in all these products. Some U.S. companies claim that no chemical treatment or preservatives are needed to prevent rawhide spoilage, because everything is done here—that is, more quickly. But many skeptics disagree, and many people no longer buy these chewies. If you do decide to give a rawhide chew to your dog, buy a high-grade product made in your own country.

Along with rawhide, three other dog treats are potentially dangerous. Smoked products are baked in giant ovens and preserved with a liquid smoke distillate that makes the bones smell "barbecued." Wood smoke contains some two hundred compounds, some of which are carcinogenic. Even for humans, keeping smoked meats to a minimum is sane advice. Second, plastic chew toys are made of petrochemical polymers such as polyurethane and nylon. No studies have been conducted to show long-term health risks for dogs, but as writer Roger Govier asks, why does one of the products include chicken if it is not meant to be eaten? On another plastic chew product, he found the words, "No added plastic, salt, sugar, color additives or preservatives." So does the product contain plastic or not? Read those labels closely, always.[25] Finally, items such as pig's ears and noses are processed with chemicals and are dyed. Many are sold in unmarked bins at big stores, which is technically illegal: according to the Food and Drug Administration (FDA), these products ought to be identified by brand, contents, and maker's address.

So what should you do when your dog gets that doggy urge to chew? Govier recommends real raw bones, carefully monitored. A few commercial chews are better than others. Try products from Doctors Foster and Smith, New England Serum Company, Pet Factory, and Ecology Rawhide Treats, made from free-range, hormone- and toxin-free cattle hides.[26]

The FDA recently issued an alert on the potential presence of salmonella in meat-based dog chews. Canadian authorities traced approximately thirty cases of salmonella to pork- or beef-based dog chews such as pig's ears and chew hooves. As a result, the big chain store PETsMART is currently investigating all the suppliers of its 570-plus superstores and will purchase only from manufacturers "that pass inspection, and test and certify that each lot is free of salmonella before shipping." The megacompany also advises you to handle the meat-based dog chews safely, treating them as if you were "preparing a chicken dinner for your family."[27]

CAT LITTER

Cats are generally fastidious and often finicky. One of their major concerns is cat litter. Is it just the right type? Is the litter box situated in the right place? Is the litter clean enough? Do they like its scent? Cats do not suffer a slightly dirty bathroom gladly. Consequently, house soiling (and the attendant odors) is the top behavioral complaint among cat guardians.

Cat litter was invented by Edward Lowe in 1947. Before he introduced his clay pellet product, breeders and cat guardians had difficulty disguising the concentrated, pungent urine of their cats. Lowe suggested a friend try a sack of pellets, which at that time were generally used to soak up oil spills on factory floors. He delivered the first hand-lettered bag of Kitty Litter to a South Bend, Indiana, pet store in 1947 and sold his company forty-three years later for more than $200 million.[28]

In the past several years, due to cats' and people's needs, cat litter options have dramatically increased. At least fifteen new varieties are now available on grocery store shelves in the United States. Consumers are becoming more concerned with convenience, and they are more aware of ingredients as well. Many consumers have more than one cat; many do not want dust fumes or wet little feet tracking dust. And they have heard the stories about cat litter causing health problems.

There are two major problems with many clay-based and clumping litters. The two ingredients in the majority of them are sodium bentonite and quartz silica (sand). Both have led to diseases and to deaths.

Sodium bentonite is often added as a clumping agent to traditional cat litters to create the "scoopable" clay litters on the market. Marina Michaels, a writer and cat breeder, refers to an article in *Cat Fancy* magazine, "How Cat Litter Is Made," in which the writers explain that sodium bentonite acts like an expandable cement, which is why these litters should not be flushed. They swell to fifteen to eighteen times their dry size and can be used as grouting, sealing, and plugging materials. If they can block a home's plumbing if flushed, what does that imply for a cat's or a rabbit's plumbing?[29]

Michaels, a breeder of Japanese bobtail cats, has lost cats in ways related to sodium bentonite. Cats not only use their litter box, they lick themselves after using it. They can thus ingest pieces of the litter. In addition, some cats sleep in their litter box and then lick their bodies. If litter gets inside a kitten or cat, it expands just as it does in the plumbing, "forming a mass and coating the interior—thus, both causing dehydration by drawing fluids out of the cat or kitten, and compounding the problem by preventing any absorption of nutrients or fluids." Michaels's cats' stools showed the color of the litter and had the consistency, smell, and texture of its clay. Another breeder she knew used a clumping litter; her veterinarian found that her kittens' lungs were coated with the litter's dust. Even though, after discovering problems, Michaels switched her kittens to a plant-based litter, she lost two of her females. Both passed clay stools until the day they died. Another kitten still passed clay almost two weeks after being switched to a new product.[30]

Michaels notes that it is not just cats that suffer health problems from these litters. So do rabbits, because they also groom themselves fervently. According to her research for the United Kingdom's House Rabbit Society, rabbit deaths have been reported due to clumping, scoopable cat litters since before 1988. In fact, the society noted that some autopsies showed that the rabbits' intestines had been cut by this substance as it tried to pass through. It warns that these clumping litters will often lead to death. Ferrets, too, are susceptible to nose blockages and possible death from clumping litters.[31]

Quoting from a study on bentonite performed by the Hennepin Center for Poison Control in Minnesota, Michaels notes that a cat known to have ingested bentonite-containing cat litter was brought to a veterinarian for lethargy and weakness. The cat was hypokalemic and anemic. Radiography revealed a small mass of radiopaque material in the cat's colon. The report notes that poisoning from the chronic ingestion of such a substance has also been reported in humans.[32]

The other toxic substance used in many cat litters is quartz silica (sand), also used in the fabrication of stone and clay products, glass, ceramic products, and more. Silica content is the reason why litters are so dusty when poured, stirred, and emptied. The International Agency for Research on Cancer has said that crystalline silica in the form of quartz or cristobalite from occupational sources should be classified as carcinogenic to humans. The group points to a large number of human studies that show its carcinogenicity when inhaled. In many of these studies lung cancer risks were increased; no other factors explained these increases. The risk of developing silicosis (which quarry workers also get from years of exposure to the dust) depends on the concentration of the crystalline silica, its particle size, and how long you are exposed. Another agency, the U.S. National Toxicology Program, describes crystalline silica (in respirable size) as a substance that "may reasonably be anticipated to be a carcinogen."[33]

Many alternative litters are now available, including pulverized cedar, a mixture of corncobs and pulverized cedar, and cedar and pine shavings. (The House Rabbit Society warns, however, that cedar and pine shavings can be dangerous.) The pressed, pelletized form of newspaper litter has no dust, which is important to small animals. Another new product is a biodegradable litter made of crystals that hold the ammonia odor especially well. Harvest Ventures of Bonifacious, Minnesota, makes this litter; Crystal Clear Litter Pearls consists of multiporous pearls that absorb odor and moisture. Several other new litters feature vegetable or tree substances, pine sawdust, or 100 percent organic corncobs. Many are compostable, flushable, and biodegradable; some feature natural odor control.

FLEA PRODUCTS

Most cats and dogs develop flea or tick problems at some time during the year. Here in northern Vermont, our cats and dog generally get them in the summertime, and they linger into fall. Fleas are a health hazard to humans and other creatures. They may transmit diseases and parasites such as tapeworms. Large numbers of fleas can also be responsible for great loss of blood, especially in young or elderly animals.

I have always had difficulty deciding what to treat our pets with, because so many of the products seem to be so toxic. As with many animal products, these are things I would not use on myself and do not want to put on my animals. However, when we tried adding garlic and brewer's yeast to their diets two years ago as an alternative to commercial flea products, we found it didn't keep the fleas away. When we have a mild year, we do little except brush, check for fleas almost daily, and maybe shampoo lightly with an organic product.

The options available in the marketplace for heavier infestations include a variety of powders, pills, collars, and injectable substances. Then there are shampoos—our second option, in the form of a "natural" substance with no obviously dangerous chemicals. Many pet stores offer flea dips here in Vermont in the summer months, which work to a varying degree depending on the fleas' tenacity.

One of the most popular new products in my area of northern Vermont of late—and, I suspect, elsewhere—has been Frontline Top-Spot. This liquid is applied to the skin between the animal's shoulder blades; it is supposed to last for a month. Its promotional materials say it is gentle enough to be used on puppies and kittens. It contains fipronil, which dissolves into the natural oils of the animal's skin and coat and works its way over the entire body. The 1999 container reads, "Active ingredient, fipronil, 9.7% for both dogs and cats, and 90.3% inert ingredients." (It also says, "Keep out of reach of children; caution.") Apparently, even if the pet goes swimming or running through puddles, the product stays in her skin. The company also offers an alcohol-based spray and recommends wearing gloves while applying its products.[34]

In a 1996 report from the New York State Department of Environmental Conservation, Division of Solid and Hazardous Materials, regarding registration of the pesticide products by Frontline, technical fipronil is found to be "moderately toxic to laboratory animals by the oral, inhalation and dermal routes of exposure . . . and mildly irritating to skin and eyes." At low doses, technical fipronil caused a number of toxicological effects in tests on rats, dogs, and rabbits. The EPA "indicated concern about chronic risks to commercial pet groomers"; the New York report, too, notes that Frontline Spray Treatment "appears to pose a great exposure potential to commercial pet groomers"—more than other products. Still, the report continues, "With regard to pet toxicity, we did not identify any significant concerns regarding toxicity to pets from use of any of the three products."[35]

The American Pet Products Manufacturers Association has estimated that 54 percent of cat owners buy flea control products. Lots of conventional veterinarians believe that the most recent products work the best. However, many are expensive and must be purchased at a veterinarian's office. Other common commercial insecticides come in several categories: botanicals, pyrethroids, carbamates, organochlorides, organophosphates, and growth regulators. The organophosphates seem to be the most toxic.[36]

Cats and Fleas

According to Jill A. Richardson, D.V.M., veterinary poison information specialist for the American Society for the Prevention of Cruelty to Animals (ASPCA) and National Animal Poison Control Center, caution must always be used when administering flea products to cats, because they are generally more sensitive to most insecticides than dogs. She warns that all products should be used exactly as indicated on the labels. She also advises:

+ Never use such products on very young kittens, pregnant queens, or debilitated or elderly cats before you consult your veterinarian.

+ Always read the instructions completely before using any such products. Do not use products on cats that are specified to be for dogs only. Some dog products can be deadly for cats, even when used in minuscule amounts.

+ Cats are more sensitive to organophosphate insecticides than most other animals. Most cat flea products do not include these as active ingredients, but many household sprays or dog products contain them. If a cat is exposed to these, she could begin drooling and suffer depression, labored breathing, weakness, and convulsions. Exposures to this substance could even lead to death.

+ Do not use flea control products that contain permethrin on cats, unless the product says it is safe. Some dog products contain high concentrations (up to 60 percent) of permethrin, and are safe on dogs but not on cats. Cats who are exposed to this can develop seizures and may tremble for days. "The fatality rate of untreated cats exposed to such products is very high," writes Dr. Richardson.

+ Be careful when using flea shampoos, sprays, or other products near your cat's eyes, ears, or genitalia. These sensitive tissues are more liable to become irritated.

+ If you use a fogger or other spray, remove all cats from the house for the time period specified on the container. Also, remove food and water bowls. Open windows or use fans to freshen the household before they return. Fumes can be irritating to your cat's eyes and to her upper respiratory system.

+ If you choose to use insect growth regulators such as lufenuron, methoprene, and pyriproxyfen, they may be used alone or in combination with over-the-counter flea control products.

+ Not all products that say "natural" are entirely safe. For example, d-limonene and linalool are citrus extracts used as flea control agents. They can still have serious side effects for some cats, however.

✦ Observe your cat closely after you use a flea product. If her behavior is different than usual, consult your veterinarian.

Richardson also warns of flea and tick collars that contain the organophosphate diazinon. These should not be used on Persian cats, in particular. This breed appears to lack the liver enzyme necessary to metabolize this substance.[37]

According to E. Kathryn Meyer, V.M.D., coordinator of the U.S. Pharmacopoeia Veterinary Practitioners' Reporting Program, which identifies medication problems and adverse reactions to drugs or chemicals, some "spot-on" flea and tick products can cause serious health problems in cats. Products that contain concentrated permethrin (45 to 65 percent) are approved for use on dogs but can be highly toxic to cats. The sprays intended for cats contain lower concentrations of permethrin (about 2 percent) and are better tolerated. Dr. Meyer's program received eleven reports between August 1997 and September 1998 involving twelve cats that needed to be hospitalized as a result of exposure to spot-on flea products. Four did not survive. Her office also received one report of a cat becoming ill merely through contact with two dogs in her household who were treated with this product. The EPA has also received reports involving 125 cats who became ill or died following the incorrect application of permethrin; 24 cats were taken sick or died because of contact with dogs treated with permethrin in their homes. In several cases animal guardians thought that a "small amount" would not harm their cats.

Meyer has called for labeling changes on such products: "These changes could include stronger warnings against the use on cats—with a description of the potentially fatal consequences of exposure—and explicit directions on how to prevent secondary exposure to cats when the product is used on dogs." If your cat suffers such toxicity, quickly bathing the feline in a mild dishwashing detergent and immediately seeking veterinary help will increase her chance of survival.[38]

Flea Pills for Dogs

In the 1990s a flea pill called Program was developed for dogs over the age of six weeks. Given once a month, it is available only through veterinarians. The dosage is based on the dog's weight. Its active ingredient is lufenuron, which breaks the flea's life cycle by inhibiting egg development. This pill has no effect on adult fleas. The tablets were tested in more than forty breeds of dogs, including pregnant females, breeding males, and puppies older than six weeks. In controlled clinical trials involving 151 dogs, the tablets provided 99 percent control of flea egg development for thirty-two days following a single dose of lufenuron at ten milligrams per kilogram of body weight. When the treatment was begun prior to the flea season, mean flea counters were lower in the Program-treated dogs than in those not treated. After six monthly treatments, the mean number of fleas (those fleas can be mean!) on Program-treated dogs was approximately 4, compared to 230 on those treated with placebos. No adverse conditions were noted.[39]

A Program flea treatment has been developed for cats in the form of an oral suspension mixed into the cat's food monthly. As for dogs, the dosage is based on the weight of the animal. Dr. Raditic notes that she is not comfortable with the idea of flea treatments taken internally, but sometimes a flea problem allows little choice.[40]

Alternatives to Chemical Flea and Tick Products

So what are your options for flea and tick control if you do not wish to use sprays, pills, or injections? Several healthy alternatives do exist. Richard Pitcairn, D.V.M., lists some of these in his book:

+ Apply herbal flea powder "sparingly" to your pet's coat.
+ Use herbal flea collars.
+ Apply natural skin tonic as a general skin toner, parasite repellent, and mange treatment.
+ Add nutritional or brewer's yeast and garlic to the animal's diet.
+ Treat your carpets with a special antiflea mineral salt.
+ Occasionally (once or twice a year) sprinkle natural, unrefined diatomaceous earth (which kills insects) along your walls, under your furniture, and in cracks where you cannot vacuum, but not directly on your animals.
+ Use sprays or powders containing pyrethrins or natural pyrethrums, which are the least toxic of all insecticides used on pets.[41]

Martin Goldstein, D.V. M., always recommends garlic and brewer's yeast, because both exude odors or tastes not attractive to fleas. Besides feeding these to your pets, he recommends sprinkling brewer's yeast on their coats every couple of days. He is also partial to Dietary Pest Control (Biovet), a powered mix of natural ingredients that is sprinkled into an animal's food. Another product he finds effective is herbal collars containing herbal flea oil made up of pennyroyal, eucalyptus, and citronella. He also uses this same oil to spray both the animals and the house.[42]

As have many veterinarians, health writer Pat Lazarus highly recommends cleaning up the animals' surrounding environment. If you have rid the fleas from your dog but they return, you may have to get fleas out of the house by vacuuming rugs, cleaning up the beds, and ridding the house of excess hair and other debris. One of Lazarus's sources, Michael Lemmon, D.V.M., also recommends cleaning with 20 Muleteam Borax or Flea Busters. These two agents—which are basically made of boron, an essential nutrient—are relatively nontoxic.[43]

Another gentle weapon against fleas is a good flea comb with tightly spaced teeth. Your pet should be combed frequently during flea season, probably every day. When you find fleas, drop them into a bucket of soap suds to kill them and stop their spread. There are also some all-natural, preservative-free foods that are good remedies for or preventors of fleas: along with brewer's yeast, try raw garlic, zinc, and barley grass concentrates. Check with your veterinarian regarding the proper dosages depending on weight. Natural repellents do exist. Essential oils such as citronella, tea tree, wintergreen, and eucalyptus have been shown to work, according to John Heinerman, author of *Natural Pet Cures: The Definitive Guide to Natural Remedies for Dogs and Cats*. He also recommends vacuuming all surfaces where fleas and their eggs may live, and washing blankets and sheets in hot water.[44]

Another product recommended by Marion Moses, M.D., director of the Pesticide Education Center, a nonprofit group in San Francisco, is a nontoxic flea control product such as Not Nice to Fleas. Nontoxic shampoos are also appropriate for both children and pets. The Pesticide Education Center can be reached at (415) 665–4722.[45]

ANIMAL COMPANIONS AS SENTINELS
OF HUMAN CANCER RISKS

Just as I was going to press with the first edition of this book, I ran across a fascinating and relevant journal article that I must include here. It covers many of the ideas previously discussed in this chapter. Titled "An Alternative Approach for Investigating the Carcinogenicity of Indoor Air Pollution: Pets as Sentinels of Environmental Cancer Risk," it was written by John A. Bukowski and Daniel Wartenberg and published in *Environmental Health Perspectives* in December 1997. In it, the authors consider the history of pet epidemiology (originally dealing with farm animals), which looks at residential cancer risk to humans by examining companion dogs' "naturally" occurring cancers. For example, researchers have noted that the prevalence of tonsillar carcinoma in dogs in the Philadelphia area is eight times higher than in dogs in rural Washington State. Other investigators found a higher risk for lymphoma in dogs exposed to electromagnetic fields near their homes. Several scientists have shown that canine and human mammary cancers share "clinical and histological features"; cigarette smoke, too, causes similar histologic changes in people's and in beagles' lungs. Radon has caused lung cancer in laboratory dogs at levels similar to those reported for uranium miners. Such observational studies of animal companion populations "represent a humane alternative to laboratory animal experimentation," and most animal guardians are more than willing to participate in such studies. "Pet dogs form an excellent surrogate population for exploring the carcinogenic potential of the domestic environment in which people live," write Bukowski and Wartenberg.[46]

6   Drinking Water

All animals need water in their diets. It affects their metabolism, their energy and mood, and their overall health. An arresting example of the effect of a lack of water is that a working dog will be 50 percent less efficient if denied it.[1]

Animals need water because it acts as a universal solvent, dissolving most chemicals in the body. If an animal or person does not drink enough water, biochemical processes do not work properly. Nutrients cannot be digested and brought to the cells, waste products are not eliminated, heat cannot be dissipated, and organs do not function as they should. The body can try to conserve water by making the urine more concentrated and by reabsorbing fluid from the feces, but this does not work well and death could occur.[2]

According to Bruce Fogle, D.V.M., "Dogs can suffer irreversible body dehydration and damage if [water] is unavailable for over 48 hours. Although canned dog food is usually three-quarters liquid, this is not enough to satisfy a dog's needs."[3] If the dog has a high temperature, is getting lots of exercise, or has a condition such as lactation, diarrhea, or other diseases, she may need more water. Approximately one ounce of water per pound of body weight per day is appropriate; if your dog is drinking three or more times this amount, she may have a disease such as diabetes or kidney failure. Bring her promptly to the veterinarian.[4] Regarding a cat's need for water, Terri McGinnis, D.V.M., writes in *The Well Cat Book*, "A cat can go without food for days and lose 30 percent to 40 percent of his or her normal body weight without dying, but a water loss of 10 percent to 15 percent can be fatal. When cats stop eating (as they do frequently when sick) they must drink more water" to offset the decreased amount of food.[5]

The rule of thumb for veterinarians is that an animal needs one milliliter of water for every food calorie consumed. For an adult cat, this means approximately 250 to 350 milliliters a day, or about 9 to 12 fluid ounces. Wet canned foods provide some water (they are approximately 78 percent water—a 6-ounce can may contain as much as 130 milliliters), but all animals also need a clean, sufficient supply of water at all times. Dry food only has about 10 percent water, so if this is all your animals eat, they need more fresh water.[6]

Yet even something as straightforward and part of everyday life as drinking water can be a culprit contributing to the development of cancer. Many pet owners now use either distilled or filtered water in their pets' dishes instead of tap water. Why? Dangerous heavy metals may make their way from the water pipes into your drinking glass or into your pet's bowl. You may inadvertently be bringing your pet closer to cadmium, copper, or lead poisoning, writes Pat Lazarus in *Keeping Your Dog Healthy the Natural Way*. A high degree of these metals in an animal's body—or in your own—can cause kidney damage, emphysema, heart disease, miscarriages, depression, and more.[7]

FLUORIDE

A potentially dangerous factor in most cities' water, added purposefully to our drinking supply, is fluoride. Since the 1940s fluoride has been an additive in toothpaste and in public drinking supplies to help prevent tooth decay. In the past twenty years tooth decay has indeed been reduced by as much as 50 percent, although the rate of reduction for this decay is lower today than it was in the 1950s. In the United States the EPA does limit the maximum concentration of fluoride in public drinking water.[8] But Pat Lazarus notes that medical studies of insects, mice, and humans have shown increased percentages of cancer caused by this additive. In an animal study performed by the National Toxicology Program (NTP), a rare liver cancer showed up in both male and female mice, and fluoride was shown to have mutagenic properties (capable of causing genetic mutations). Although the NTP did not report all its conclusions, in an

EPA evaluation of its tests Dr. William L. Marcus (then chief toxicologist for the EPA's drinking water program) said that three out of four in vitro tests proved fluoride to be mutagenic, "supporting the conclusion that fluoride is a probable human carcinogen."[9] In a report in *The Ecologist* a journal of the United Kingdom, is this admission, "It [fluoride] has even been blamed by doctors from the United States' National Cancer Institute and National Health Federation for 35,000 cancer deaths every year."[10]

Amazingly, in the United Kingdom the minister of state for public health, Tessa Jowell, has been proposing for several years to give health authorities the power to compel water companies to fluoridate all water for the purpose of dental hygiene. According to a 2004 statement from the British Anti-Vivisection Association, "Tessa Jowell, 'Minister for Public Health', knowing that there is NO evidence showing that fluoride reduces tooth decay, and having been shown conclusive evidence that the chemical is a major threat to health, is still pushing for a fluoride-poisoned nation."[11] Fluoridation has already been rejected in Belgium, Norway, France, the Czech Republic, and Austria.

In health-related studies, several trials using mice, rats, and rabbits have shown that long-term ingestion of sodium fluoride adversely affects the fertility of the males. On-going fluoride intake has also been linked to lowered human birth rates and to decreased amounts of testosterone. "In vitro exposure of human sperm to fluoride produced a significant decline in sperm motility."[12]

Lazarus quotes Dean Burk, a former researcher at the U.S. Public Health Service's National Cancer Institute, as saying, "Our data in the United States indicate in my view that one-tenth of all cancer deaths in this country can be shown to be linked to fluoridation of public drinking water. . . . [That] exceeds deaths from breast cancer."[13]

CHLORINE

And of course, there is chlorine in many water supplies. Chlorine was added to public water as an effective disinfectant in the early 1900s; as a result, typhoid fever, cholera, and dysentery almost disappeared in the United States. But chlorine has also been linked to various cancers. A Finnish study indicates that MX, a compound formed when chlorine reacts with organic material in water, causes cancer in lab rats when they swallow large amounts of it. "MX should be studied as a candidate risk factor," the Finnish scientists conclude.[14]

What most concerns many scientists about chlorine are its by-products, called trihalomethanes or THMs. Risks of various human cancers are being correlated to the use of chlorinated drinking water. Some research indicates that the incidence of cancer is 44 percent higher among those who drink chlorinated water. For example, cancers of the kidney, bladder, and urinary tract are common in certain U.S. cities, such as New Orleans, which gets its tap water from the Mississippi River and adds large amounts of chlorine to protect against infectious disease. According to one report, "Approximately 63 new carcinogenic compounds are created in Mississippi drinking water when chlorine combines with methanol, carbon disulphide, and other substances." The President's Council on Environmental Quality (established by the U.S. Congress in 1969) has said, "There is increased evidence for an association between rectal, colon and bladder cancer and the consumption of chlorinated drinking water."[15]

Cold drinking water generally contains the highest concentration of THMs because it is drunk straight from the kitchen tap. Hot beverages have lower THM levels because of volatilization from heating; so do cold beverages that are stored for long periods in open containers.[16] Such storage will also evaporate most chlorine by-products.

MTBE

MTBE is methyl tertiary-butyl ether, a chemical that helps gasoline burn clean. It is an oxygenate, an octane booster that is blended into gas. In the United States alone 4.5 billion gallons a year are produced. A U.S. law requires its presence in gasoline. The problem it creates for drinking water exists because gas stations sometimes experience leaks, resulting in gas moving through the groundwater and into well water.

According to many authorities, 20 percent of U.S. urban wells now have some MTBE. It is the second most common water contaminant in the country. In California alone the chemical is found in the groundwater of some ten thousand sites; it is found in some amounts in forty-nine states. The TV program *60 Minutes* has discussed a study in which cancer was created in lab animals when MTBE was administered in high levels. In another study performed five years ago in Italy, MTBE caused high rates of lymphoma, testicular cancer, and leukemia in lab rats.[17]

According to a report in *Chemical Market Report,* in April 1999 the East Coast used 130,000 barrels of MTBE daily; the West Coast, 100,000 barrels a day, representing the highest usages in the country.[18] In one town, Glenville, California, the town and government discovered MTBE in the water supply in August 1997. The residents can no longer use it for drinking or cooking. Many have intestinal problems and skin rashes, and the majority of businesses have closed. Glenville is now practically a ghost town. All this from one leak at one gas station.

In 1999, the EPA was "urging a prompt nationwide phaseout of methyl tertiary butyl ether in reformulated gasoline, following an advisory panel's conclusion."[19] In mid-March 2000, the EPA announced should Congress fail to agree on a way to phase MTBE out of gasoline, "that it [the EPA] would move toward a ban" of the additive, which was "expected to take as long as three years to become paractice."[20] However, in April 2005 the House of Representatives voted "to shield makers of the gasoline additive MTBE from lawsuits involving the contamination of drinking water." According to Rep. Lois Capps, D-Calif., "groundwater contamination from the gasoline additive has affected more than 1,800 community water systems in 29 states." More than eighty lawsuits have been filed. The new bill, however, does call for "phasing out MTBE use by the end of 2014," some twelve years longer than originally anticipated.[21]

OTHER TOXIC CHEMICALS

Richard Pitcairn, D.V.M., warns that fluoride is only one of more than twenty-one hundred toxic chemicals that have been detected in U.S. water. A few of the others are lead, cadmium, arsenic, toluene, and nitrates. Many of these pollutants are known to cause cancer or damage the kidneys, liver, brain, and cardiovascular system. Communities with highly polluted water display high rates of gastrointestinal and urinary organ cancer. People who have drunk only chlorinated water over their lifetimes have a higher rate of bladder cancer and possibly of colon and rectal cancers. Dr. Pitcairn and his coauthor, Susan Hubble Pitcairn, recommend a good-quality water purifier. They also stress the importance of changing your pet's water daily. Keep the bowl clean and in a clean, uncluttered place. I wash our pets' water bowls at least weekly. Your pets should always be able to reach a water bowl with clean water so they will not be tempted to drink out of puddles, creeks, or ponds, which may be contaminated.[22]

DRINKING BOWLS

Speaking of water bowls, the healthiest materials to use are (most) ceramics and stoneware, glass, or stainless steel. Stainless steel works well because its surface does not absorb odors, stain, corrode, or rust. Stoneware dishes are recommended by a variety of sources, including Doctors Foster and Smith, a dog and cat product supplier. This supplier indicates that studies show cats drink more water from pottery dishes than they do from metal or plastic ones, decreasing the incidence of another cat disease, feline urological syndrome (FUS).[23] Also, the animals cannot chew the bowl or pick it up, reducing spillage.

Whatever its material, your bowl of choice should be able to be scalded with boiling water for cleaning, be large enough for your animal to enjoy, and be steady enough that it does not tip over easily.[24]

THE HEALTHIEST WATER

Pat Lazarus recommends that if you wish to continue using tap water, be sure to let it run for five minutes before you use it. This will help rid the water of eroded heavy metal from your pipes, providing a partial solution. However, Lazarus strongly recommends buying a water filter that you can attach to your faucet. Read the fine print, though; some filters eliminate more contaminants than others.

If you decide on a filter for your own and your animals' drinking water, choose one carefully. There are substantial differences. According to information from the Environmental Health Program, part of Health Canada's Health Protection branch, the filter should contain activated carbon and should be properly maintained. Filters can themselves become sources of bacterial contamination.

In the veterinary community (and I suspect the human medical community as well), there is currently a controversy about the advantages of springwater over distilled water. Pat Lazarus has found that most holistic veterinarians prefer distilled water, because they feel springwater is often contaminated. Distilled water leaches minerals out of the body, but these are "undesirable, inorganic" minerals. Some holistic veterinarians even use distilled water as one therapy for arthritis in dogs, because it does rid these undesirable minerals from the animals' bodies.[25]

If you decide to stick with tap water, do keep an eye on your pet's water dish. If it begins to show discoloration, consider your tap water the culprit—and change the dish. In a case study Lazarus included in one of her books, *Healing the Mind the Natural Way,* a woman and her dog developed similar psychosomatic symptoms; the woman's symptoms did not respond to various psychological therapies. At the same time, discoloration of the dog's water bowl led her to have her water pipes tested. She found that they had many times the safe level of copper in their household pipes. She and the puppy both had copper poisoning; both were cured by nutritional doctors (and, presumably, by finding a different source of water).[26]

Trying to make sure your drinking water supply is safe for both you and your pets is tricky. Susan W. Putnam and Jonathan Baert Wiener write, "Efforts to reduce one risk in drinking water may introduce—either intentionally or unintentionally—a different risk to the population using the water supply. . . . This dilemma is at the core of modern drinking water policy." They state that there is no simple solution regarding assessing the risks and advantages of local drinking water. But, they add, "We need to weigh all of the risks of drinking water in a thoughtful, sensible manner and search for solutions that reduce overall risk."[27]

One final note regarding hard versus soft water: Hard water contains high amounts of dissolved minerals, including calcium and magnesium. This varies by region and generally poses no serious health concerns for a healthy animal. However, there have been human cases of calcium-based bladder stones resulting from drinking a lot of hard water. A water-softening system is probably a good idea. Soft water, by contrast, often replaces minerals such as calcium and magnesium with sodium. However, the amount of sodium in this soft water is small compared to that in cat foods. Still, for people or animals with any heart disease, this additional sodium could be burdensome in the process of monitoring and restricting sodium in the diet.[28]

7 Nutrition

One of the most critical pieces of the cancer puzzle is food. Certainly, if you are reading this book, you already probably know quite a bit about nutrition for your animals. You have probably bought at least one of the dozens of new books that have appeared over the past decade extolling the benefits of natural foods and even some raw foods for our animal companions. Because so much literature is available on pet food in the marketplace, I will not cover it exhaustively in this book. Suffice it to say, however, that proper nutrition may be the most important factor in keeping your animals healthy—both for prevention against diseases such as cancer *and* for maintaining their immune systems during any treatments for cancer.

In the spring of 1998 a survey of attitudes toward animal nutrition was mailed to seven hundred veterinarian and student members of the Association of Veterinarians for Animal Rights. Although only one hundred fifty replied, their responses are telling. Eighty percent of the respondents believe that nutrition should be part of therapy for dogs with cancer. Nearly 79 percent believe that nutrition therapy is important for cats with cancer. More than 65 percent answered "definitely yes" to the question "Do you believe a qualitative difference exists among commercial pet food brands?" and more than 68 percent believe that pet food companies do not provide adequate information about their products. Only approximately 20 percent frequently advised home cooking for healthy cats and dogs, but more than 32 percent did so for the treatment of health problems. A few of the most telling comments were as follows: "I think that it is long overdue that pet food companies are investigated for the ingredients placed in pet food"; "Nutrition is the future and the only hope for preventing and curing disease"; and "Nutrition is the most overlooked and probably the most important aspect of all medicine."[1]

And not only veterinarians believe in the primacy of nutrition in animal health. As one natural pet food manufacturer says succinctly, "Nutrition, not breed, is the single most limiting factor to your pet's health and longevity."[2] We all know by now that the route to travel is not the one down the grocery store's aisles. But what about the other high-quality "natural" dog and cat foods?

THE PET FOOD INDUSTRY

Perhaps the most shocking and informative book about the pet food industry is Ann Martin's *Food Pets Die For,* published in 1997. As Dr. Michael W. Fox, vice president of the Humane Society of the United States, says, "Ann Martin is to the pet food industry what Rachel Carson was to the petro-chemical-pesticide industry."[3] Martin spent seven years investigating the commercial pet food industry, and what she uncovered isn't pretty.

There are several reasons you really do not want to feed your dog or cat commercial foods only. Perhaps the most compelling reason, morally, is that there are rendered, euthanized pets in much of this food. These pets have been mixed with other materials, including some condemned for human foods: "rotten meat from supermarket shelves, restaurant grease . . . '4-D' (dead, diseased, dying, and disabled) animals, roadkill." The Minister of Agriculture of Québec told Martin that, indeed, dead animals are cooked with viscera, bones, and fats; the fur is not removed. In both the United States and Canada, this rendering of animal companions is not illegal. Martin points to an article originally published in the *San Francisco Chronicle* in which an employee and ex-employee of a rendering plant admitted that their company rendered approximately 250,000 to 500,000 pounds of animals, scraps, and more, including "somewhere between 10,000 and 30,000 pounds of dogs and cats a day."[4]

That's enough to put most of us off, isn't it? Martin, a Canadian writer who lives with several animal companions, went a bit further in her investigations and discovered that some animals are euthanized with sodium pentobarbital and then rendered. This does not break down the poison, yet this rendered material goes into commercial pet food and into feed for cows, pigs, and horses.[5]

Richard Pitcairn, D.V.M., states that fewer than one out of every quarter million animals slaughtered in this country "is tested for toxic chemical residues."[6] Martin adds that a pet food manufacturer *might* reject some rendered materials for a variety of reasons: these include "off odor . . . excessive feathers . . . bone chunks . . . added blood . . . heavy metals . . . insect infestation" and more.[7]

Wendell O. Belfield, D.V.M., author of *How to Have a Healthier Dog* and *The Very Healthy Cat Book* (both written with Martin Zucker), was a veterinary meat inspector for the USDA and the state of California for seven years. He saw terrible things in this job, including the use of dead pets with sodium pentobarbital in their bodies. In the finished rendered products, fat stabilizers are introduced to prevent rancidity. BHA and BHT are "both known to cause liver and kidney dysfunction." Some European countries prohibit their use or importation. Ethoxyquin (EQ) is "suspected of being a cancer-causing agent." Many semimoist dog foods contain propylene glycol, a cousin of antifreeze that "causes the destruction of red blood cells." Dr. Belfield informs us that lead often shows up in pet foods, too, simply as a result of our environment. Pulling no punches, Belfield concludes, "Any veterinary nutritionist, government health official, or scientist who says feeding the aforementioned chemicals daily to our pets will not have a deleterious effect on them is living in a fool's paradise."[8]

According to a brochure put out by the Ralston Purina Company, certain information is required on all pet food packages, including "crude protein (minimum amount); crude fat (minimum amount); crude fiber (maximum amount), and moisture (maximum amount)." The word *crude* means that the amounts are determined by laboratory trials. While these trials "can verify that the guaranteed nutrients are in the diet, these components may not be available to the pet." The nutritional adequacy should instead be determined by feeding trials, I believe, and should be labeled thus. However, note that even products with labels saying "feeding tests" or something similar may not have gone through feeding tests; they may be part of a "family" of products that underwent the trials.

The Ralston Purina brochure goes on to say that all ingredients in pet food "must be listed on the label in descending order of predominance by weight." If the product is not nutritionally complete or balanced, the label must say so with a disclaimer such as "not to be fed as a sole diet" to protect consumers. A product named, for instance, "beef dinner" must contain at least 10 percent beef, and beef must be listed in the ingredients. A designation such as "with cheese" guarantees only 3 percent of the particular ingredient.

But even the Ralston Purina brochure admits that labels do not tell us everything we need to know. "It is necessary to rely on the manufacturer's testing, research and overall reputation to ensure that the pet food is of high quality." The company recommends contacting the manufacturer or distributor if you have questions regarding ingredients in your dog's or cat's daily food products.[9]

According to the Animal Protection Institute of Sacramento, California, commercial pet foods—those sold in convenience and grocery stores—contain mostly grains and meat by-products, which may be the euthanized shelter animals mentioned above or even "cancer-ridden livestock." Federal meat inspector and veterinarian P. F. McGargle has noted that "feeding these low-in-nutrition packaged 'scraps' to pets increases their chances of cancer and other degenerative diseases." Still, more than 95 percent of our animal companions in the United States derive their primary nutrition from "processed pet foods, mostly these grocery store brands."[10]

In the United States four of the five major pet food companies are part of major multinational food production companies: Colgate-Palmolive, Heinz, Nestle, and Mars, the original pet food manufacturer. The pet food industry is actually an extension of the human food industry, although the pets get fed what we would not consider eating, that "unfit for human consumption."[11] In addition, it delivers to a large, lucrative, and growing market. As of 1995 combined sales of cat and dog foods in the United States were $9.3 billion; all categories except moist cat foods showed increases.[12]

Two-thirds of the pet food manufactured in the United States contains added preservatives, according to the Animal Protection Institute.

There are many additives as well, including coloring agents, emulsifiers, lubricants, flavoring agents, pH control agents, synergists, solvents, and a dozen or so more. "Of the more than 8,600 recognized food additives today, no toxicity information is available for 46% of them," the institute claims. "Cancer-causing agents are sometimes permitted if they are used at low enough levels."[13] The buildup of these agents certainly must be deleterious to our animal companions' health and happiness.

Three common preservatives in pet foods, BHA, BHT, and EQ, have been shown to lead to development of certain cancers. BHA and BHT are the most common antioxidants in processed food for humans. The Animal Protection Institute states there is little information available to document their toxicity or safety for animals. EQ is the most common antioxidant preservative in pet foods. It has been found in some dogs' livers and tissues months after the animals stopped ingesting it. As of July 31, 1997, the FDA's Center for Veterinary Medicine requested that pet food manufacturers cut in half the maximum level for EQ.[14]

A synthetic preservative, EQ helps keep the vitamin E in food efficacious. The shelf life of products preserved only with vitamins C and E is shorter than that of products preserved with BHA or EQ. Natural antioxidants are inherently unstable, so synthetic antioxidants are used to stabilize fats and oils. But is a longer shelf life the most important quality in our nonhuman family members' food?[15]

Ethoxyquin is manufactured by Monsanto Chemical, the company best known of late as the largest manufacturer of bioengineered foods. The containers are marked POISON. EQ is listed as a hazardous chemical by the Occupational Safety and Health Administration (OSHA), and as a pesticide by the USDA.[16] It is used in most U.S. dog food but is banned in Europe. While Monsanto's own results from a required 1996 study found ethoxyquin to have no significant toxicity, "the FDA's Center for Veterinary Medicine requested that pet food manufacturer's voluntarily reduce the maximum level for ethoxyquin by half to 75 parts per million."[17]

However, not all veterinarians are worried about this preservative. Donald R. Strombeck, D.V.M., author of *Home-Prepared Dog and Cat Diets: The Healthful Alternative,* a book highly recommended to me by other veterinarians, states that ethoxyquin is "safe as well as effective.

There is more than three-quarters of a century of study of this chemical. As with almost any chemical, if a dog or cat receives enough, it can be toxic"—but the amount added to commercial pet food causes "no problems." Dr. Strombeck adds that this antioxidant, more than others, has "anticancer properties. It interferes with cancer induction by other chemicals through actions not dependent on being an antioxidant." So, as with so many issues covered in this book, there is little if any agreement within the veterinary community about the safety of EQ.[18]

One conclusion that can be drawn about commercial pet food is that, according to Ann Martin's extensive research, strict regulations of products do not exist in either the United States or Canada. "What is needed, in both the United States and Canada, are government-enforced regulations of this industry. Until then, *Buyer Beware*," she writes.[19] As of April 2004 no standards are yet in place for pet foods.[20]

DIFFERENT CATEGORIES OF COMMERCIAL FOODS

Many different types of pet foods are available in grocery stores, independent pet food stores, and megastores such as PETsMART. They fall into four categories: generic, name-brand, premium, and specialty. Generic or store-brand pet foods are less expensive and of lower quality. Generally they do not claim to be complete or balanced, and they are not. Most of us would buy them only in a pinch while traveling or in an emergency, when no pet store is open. Name-brand foods are similar to the bulk of frozen dinners you might buy at the supermarket. Writes Dr. Martin Goldstein, "We like to think that commercial brands contain at least some decent cuts of [meat or fish]. The truth is they contain none. Any cuts fit for human consumption are consumed by humans."[21] These brands are familiar and have been around for a long time. Many people still trust them.

Premium foods include Science Diet, Eukanuba, California Natural, and more. These are found in pet supply or pet specialty stores, or sometimes in your veterinarian's hospital or office. They cost more, and the manufacturers insist that the ingredients are higher quality. For example, "in a generic food you might find legs and beaks of processed chickens; in a name-brand, it might be the chicken organs;

and in the premium food, it might be the same cuts of chicken that we would eat."[22]

Then there are specialty diets, higher priced yet and labeled "natural," including Wysong, Abady, Natural Life, and more. You can find organic diets (made with organic grains, vegetables, meat, poultry, and fish, without chemicals); vegetarian diets; and prescription diets (primarily Hill's diets, which are available only through veterinarians' offices).[23] The word *natural* can mean a variety of things: it may mean the food contains no dyes or chemicals, or it may mean that the product contains no chemicals, artificial coloring, or chemical preservatives. It may also mean that it contains quality meats, fruits, vegetables, and herbs for the sake of health maintenance.[24] There appears to be no standard or verifiable definition of the use of this word in pet foods. According to even newer definitions, offered by Narda Robinson, D.V.M., in *Veterinary Practice News,* "natural means that products are minimally processed and contain no artificial ingredients. . . . Organic refers instead to how producers either grow crops or raise animals, and has specific criteria and certification parameters."[25] You must read labels carefully and question what you read. Call or write the manufacturer to ask direct questions.

Since the first edition of this book, several new pet food products are available raw or cooked and frozen in individual servings. One of the most successful—and available—of these is Steve's Real Food, made of raw meat, fruit, and vegetables, using "100% human quality ingredients." His foods consist of three parts: organ meat and muscle (60% for dogs, 81% for cats), fruits and vegetables, (38% for dogs, 15% for cats,) and a special blend of other nutrients, minerals, vitamins (2% for dogs, 4% for cats). The food amount recommended is 1½% to 2% of your animal's body weight.

His three food products are named Charlee Bear Dogs, Charlee Bear Dog Treats, and Steve's Real Food for Pets. Just this spring, 2004, he and coauthor, Beth Taylor, who teaches people how to train, exercise, and feed dogs, wrote the practical book, *See Spot Live Longer,* about feeding your dog more nutritiously to help him live a longer life. Steve Brown is a breeder of dogs he calls "perfect hybrids." One of the reasons Steve Brown wrote the book is because "my dog of all dogs, Zach, a special mixed-breed (hybrid) called a Charlee Bear Dog, died of cancer at age 10. I expected him to live to age 16." He notes, "together, we (Beth and I) have fed about 25,000 dogs."[26]

Another relatively new product is KARMA, put out by Natura Pet Products. Labeled "the first certified organic meat-based food for dogs," it is made of more than 95% organic ingredients. A few include free-range chicken, brown rice, barley, quinoa, red beets, spinach, blueberries, and green tea extract. Karma advertises that it contains 18 certified organic ingredients making it the highest percentage of any dog food on the market. The food is certified organic by Quality Assurance International under the USDA's National Organic Program guidelines. "Additionally, Karma is created in adherence with human food quality standards, thus establishing Karma as the highest quality organic food for dogs on the market."[27]

THE NUTRITION DILEMMA

Donna Raditic, D.V.M.—who did undergraduate work in animal nutrition, and is currently pursuing a three to four year study program through the American College of Veterinary Nutrition—takes her nutrition counseling seriously. She explained to me recently that the veterinary industry has changed radically over the past few decades. Veterinarians no longer treat "our food source," they treat "our family."[28] Do we really want our family to be eating harmful foods and additives on a daily basis? Many of us sneak to McDonald's once in a while, without telling anyone, perhaps when we are on a long road trip. But would we willingly eat this food daily or feed it to our human family every day?

Why then have we agreed to feed our animal companions commercially prepared foods for so long? One reason, of course, is convenience, something that many of us settle for in our rushed lives. Nick Downing, a senior analyst with Datamonitor Europe who has examined trends in the pet food industry, writes, "Longer working hours, increasing numbers of working women and the growth of single adult households have placed increasing pressure on time, creating a strong demand for easy-to-keep, 'low-maintenance' pets."[29] This is true of foods for our animals, and often for ourselves. Haven't many of us resorted to ordering pizza once a week, or using the microwave for frozen dinners (even if they are vegetarian) more often than cooking a nutritious meal of organic meat or fish, vegetables, and grains?

Coupled with this is the mounting concern many of us share about health and fitness issues—and that includes the health of our pets. Continues Downing, "The health factor has also been a crucial driving force behind today's petfood market. . . . [Consumers] are keen to ensure that their pets receive the best in terms of nutrition—fueling the growth of superpremium and nutraceutical products."[30] Most holistic or alternative veterinarians are recommending for their animal clients a homemade diet with the occasional addition of store-bought food. However, Downing concludes on this note: "New product development will reflect trends in the human food industry. . . . This is set to continue as the quality of petfood rises and the gap between human and animal food narrows."[31]

THE HOMEMADE DIET

So what *is* a healthy diet for our animals, and how can we provide it for them? Many veterinarians and nutritionists agree on what equals a healthy diet in general terms, but there are many differences of opinion regarding its actual ingredients. Raw versus cooked, bones versus no bones, organic versus nonorganic? Let's look at a few recommendations. In her book *Keep Your Dog Healthy the Natural Way*, writer Pat Lazarus recommends a homemade diet and describes the optimal preventive diet for an adult dog this way: One-third to one-half of the daily diet should be animal foods, preferably raw. These include chicken, turkey, organ meats, and occasionally fish. "Never give cooked bones, and be careful of bones in general," she writes. Sometimes other animal protein may be substituted, such as yogurt, raw milk, and raw egg yolks. Vegetables, fruits, and grains should make up most of the rest of the daily diet. The grains should be cooked; the vegetables and fruits, raw. Finally, the diet should include some polyunsaturated oil such as safflower or sesame oil; pure water; and vitamin and mineral supplements.[32]

Dr. Pitcairn, also recommends a homemade diet; his is slightly different and a bit more complex. The following basic diet works for both cats and dogs, but in different quantities. It includes a variety of meats—

hamburger, chicken, and turkey, some organ meats—mostly lean and ground up, and often fed raw. Although Pitcairn knows that many veterinarians are opposed to feeding raw meat because of concern about contracting diseases, in seventeen years of recommending raw foods he has never seen a problem with this practice. In fact, he sees improved health when animals are fed raw meat. He also includes dairy products (raw milk, cottage cheese, yogurt); eggs (either raw or lightly cooked); whole grains, cooked; legumes such as lentils, soybeans, split peas; and vegetables, ideally raw, such as carrots or alfalfa sprouts, though cooked corn, broccoli, and others can be included, all preferably organic. He also lists a lot of snacks and flavorings such as garlic and yeast sprinkles, along with supplements such as bonemeal, kelp, and several vitamins and vegetable oils.[33] His book *Dr. Pitcairn's Complete Guide to Natural Health for Dogs and Cats* lists many recipes for dogs and cats, both complex and quick; I highly recommend it.

Like most nutrition-conscious veterinarians, Dr. Pitcairn does not recommend a vegetarian diet—especially not for cats, who are carnivores. Cats clearly require nutrients supplied only by meat and animal products. The dog is more closely an omnivore—wolves and coyotes consume lots of vegetable matter—and so requires less meat. Pitcairn is concerned, however, about the quality of meat on the market and about how those feed animals are treated: "Even the highest-quality cuts approved for human consumption contain residues of antibiotics, synthetic hormones and toxic materials such as lead, arsenic, mercury, DDT and dioxin."[34] He recommends using more poultry, eggs, and dairy products than beef; turkey is preferable to chicken, because it is raised more humanely and on vegetarian feed. You *can* cut meat out of a dog's diet if she eats soy protein instead, but a diet that excludes meat is, again, not ideally suited for a cat.[35]

Some researchers disagree. According to Lorelei Wakefield, a student at the University of Pennsylvania, "Taurine is supplemented in the commercially available vegan cat foods: Evolution and VegeCat. Even regular meat-based pet food has synthetic taurine added because it's cooked at such high temperatures that much of the taurine present in the meat is destroyed," she wrote me in August 2004.[36] During the five years between this edition and the last, she and her mentor, Dr. Kathryn Michel, have performed a study on vegetarian diets for cats. The researchers looked at pet cats—thirty-four on vegetarian diets and fifty-two control cats—between June and August 2004. Lab animals were not the subjects of the study, and no invasive procedures were performed. "To date, there have not been any scientific studies about the health and nutritional status of vegetarian cats in the U.S.," state its researchers, vet student Wakefield and clinical nutritionist faculty sponsor, Dr. Michel. Nestle Purina funded the project. But at the time of this publication, the results were not yet ready. "Good science takes a long time," noted Wakefield.[37]

Dr. Raditic, who, unlike most veterinarians, has an extensive background in animal nutrition, recommends a homemade diet or the highest-quality prepared foods plus supplements. She does not advocate raw food, because she feels that most dogs and cats do not have good digestive capabilities. For animal diets, she lightly cooks vegetables, and says that white rice is more digestible for many animals than brown. She does believe that animals can sometimes eat raw eggs without harm. She also recommends a book by veterinarian Donald R. Strombeck, *Home-Prepared Dog and Cat Diets: The Healthful Alternative* (see appendix B).

In fall 2004, she added this advice, "Current thoughts in cancer nutrition include limiting simple carbohydrates in the diet as cancer cells like glucose (simple sugars) as an energy supply. These patients seem to do better on proteins, fats, and complex carbohydrate diets." She still recommends home-prepared diets or some commercially prepared raw diets for maximum success, and adds, "Omega 3 fatty acids, Vitamin A and D therapy are standing out as nutritional supplements in cancer treatments."[38]

In a 1990s study in the United Kingdom, eighty-nine owners of 126 dogs changed from feeding their pets processed pet food to giving natural bones and vegetables. Seventy-four percent of the respondents changed to the diet Ian Billinghurst, B.V.Sc., recommended in his book *Give Your Dog a Bone,* and 13 percent already fed their canines a similar diet. Billinghurst's diet is called the B. A. R. F. diet—ie., bones and raw food. After six months the respondents reported a drop of 85 percent in vet visits. Other changes included: "more energy and activity, improved teeth and gums, glossier coats, and skin, weight and behavioural improvements." The dogs also had fewer fleas, better appetites, cleaner ears, no stomach and digestive upsets, better breath, and no scratching, and they no longer required veterinary medication." The high rates (88 percent) of benefits were achieved by feeding a diet including raw chicken wings, raw meaty lamb, pork and beef bones, raw "green tripe," and both cooked and uncooked vegetables. (There is no mention of dairy, grains, or vitamin or mineral supplements in this diet.) The canines' health improvements increased over time. Even dogs on the diet for a few weeks showed improvements.[39]

Dr. Billinghurst operates a solo practice, working six to seven days a week. "Of late," he writes in December 2004, "the cancer I see in practice appears to have declined, but then a large proportion of my clients have moved away from processed food for their pets."[40] Robert McDowell, N.D., an Australian herbalist who works with many animals with cancer, highly recommends Dr. Billinghurst's diet. He has seen an alarming rise in cancer incidence in Australian dogs, and now in cats and horses. His advice? "Institute immediately the B.A.R.F. diet, possibly modified as per my discussion on natural sources of vitamins. Then settle on, and persist with, a simple program of immune system and antioxidant support along with other programs addressed to the specific type of cancer and to the health and treatment history overall."[41]

Another study, this in Sweden, compared the impact of processed, cooked food versus raw food on animals as they aged. Initially, the animals that ate the processed foods prospered. As they reached adulthood, however, they began to age more quickly than the control group, and to develop chronic degenerative disease symptoms. The control group raised on raw foods aged less quickly and did not have these diseases. Similarly, other researchers have concluded that processed pet food suppresses the immune system and can lead to heart, kidney, liver, and other diseases.[42]

Alfred J. Plechner, D.V.M., author with Martin Zucker of *Pets at Risk,* a book about treating endocrine-immune imbalances in animal companions, says the following: "I have carefully weighed the merits of raw meat versus cooked meat. I conclude that for my patients, cooked meat represents less of a chance to develop a catastrophic bacterial disease than raw meat."[43] As of this second edition, the raw food diet still is not the most popular or advised by veterinarians, although it surely has its advocates, particularly in countries other than the United States.

In other countries, the situation may be different, depending on the quality and source of the meat. Australian veterinarian Clare Middle told me that a natural diet incorporating organic or biodynamically grown vegetables and cereal could either prevent cancer or lessen the likelihood of its recurrence, considering that most veterinarians accept that chemical and pesticide residues in foods may be a factor in causing cancer. In her area kangaroo is a free-range and pesticide-free meat appropriate for animal consumption.[44]

Another Australian veterinarian, Carolyn J. Ashton, suspects that her country's commercial foods are more strictly monitored than those in the United States. She always recommends a fresh-food diet and "human quality food, not pet quality" for the higher "life vitality" in the food. She recommends raw meat but realizes that not all animals will tolerate it. She believes this better approximates their wild diet, and that cooking meat increases the absorption of proteins and their phenolic compounds as well as increasing its allergenic potential. She advocates a balanced diet that includes supplements such as omega-3 and omega-6 essential fatty acids, and nutrient powders such as lecithin, kelp, and wheat germ. Finally, she advises raw bones—with the proviso that raw lamb bones in Australia can set off pancreas inflammation (as does the marrow in marrowbones). "I never let them eat them [raw bones] unobserved though," she notes.[45]

Kymythy Schultze, a breeder of Newfoundland dogs and teacher of holistic care for dogs and cats in the state of Washington, feels that a balanced diet for dogs includes raw meat, bones, vegetables, herbs, and oils. She recommends thinking in terms of "prey animal" proportions. What ingredients might your dog find in a rabbit or a bird, for example? She contends this is in large part raw bones, and also muscle and organ meat. She recommends lots of raw meat, fish, and eggs to provide adequate protein, and cod-liver or flaxseed oil to supply essential fatty acids. She also recommends kelp to help balance the glands.[46]

THREE TYPES OF HOMEMADE DIETS

Joe Bodewes, D.V.M., lists the three kinds of homemade diets as these: "the true, well-balanced, nutritiously complete entirely homemade diet"; the supplemented homemade diet—a commercial dry food serves as at least half the diet, with added meat, some carbohydrate sources, and the family leftovers, perhaps with a multivitamin; and table food only, which the owner "doesn't balance . . . for protein, fat, carbohydrates and vitamins." Dr. Bodewes feels that the latter is not a good diet. "It is often fed to finicky eaters . . . the owner prepares a 'special' diet that may consist of chicken breast or turkey but lacks fiber, and the correct vitamins and minerals." He lists several factors to think about before going the homemade route:

+ Such a diet often takes more of your time.
+ It may be more expensive than commercial kibble.
+ It needs to be supplemented with a balanced multivitamin.
+ A homemade diet not properly balanced can be worse than a commercial diet.
+ It should not be too soft, because solid, crunchy food helps clean pets' teeth.
+ Switching over takes a period of three weeks to avoid intestinal problems.
+ Without adequate exercise, "the best diet in the world won't improve your pet's health."[47]

SWITCHING OVER

It takes a few days—if not weeks—to make any dietary switch with animals. Many veterinarians recommend switching from commercial to homemade foods gradually; you can even mix some high-quality store-bought product in with your homemade diet. Problems that may occur are diarrhea, gas, or "rumbly stomach," something our dogs have suffered.

In *The New Natural Cat*, Anita Frazier recommends giving cats just a tablespoon of the new diet at first. Some cats may nibble; others will not. Even though some animal lovers may feel Fluffy will go hungry, you can give three or four meals a day at first as long as you remove all food after half an hour. Frazier feels that 98 percent of all cats will make the switch successfully in a day. If after two days your cats will not eat the new food, she recommends a special treats ploy—mixing in "bribe foods" such as lightly cooked chicken liver or a sardine. After eight days, feed only the new diet, as much as the cat wants twice daily.[48]

THE OTHER SIDE

If you do want to go the homemade route, you should know that some experts have voiced concerns about such diets—especially if they involve raw foods. Breeders and vets who recommend raw diets point to the fact that wild dogs eat raw meat and other uncooked delights. But of course, much of the meat we buy in the grocery store is contaminated, and this can seriously upset a dog's digestive system, as it sometimes does ours. Even blanching meat may not eliminate all the harmful bacteria it contains.

Dr. Sharon Machlik, director of technical marketing for Nutro Products, maker of superpremium dog and cat foods, believes that preparing a raw diet (especially if you sprout seeds) can take quite a long time, including pureeing and cleanup. Furthermore, not all breeders know what amount of which ingredients are critical to an animal's health. For example, a high level of selenium can prove toxic to dogs. Meaty bones may provide ten to twenty times more phosphorous than calcium—far too much, in Dr. Machlik's estimation. Although she does agree that bones are a fine source of minerals, she recommends grinding them up finely. Bones can splinter and cause internal damage, or can lead to diarrhea and vomiting. They can also cause broken teeth, which will then affect a dog's ability to eat other foods. She concludes, "In my view, the raw diet for dogs is a fad, and one to be avoided by breeders and dog owners in general. Far better to leave diet preparation to those who know it best: the makers of petfood who use only high quality ingredients."[49]

DOG DIET SUGGESTIONS

If you would like to gradually improve your canine companion's diet but are not quite ready to cook a doggie stew every few days, here are a few easy changes to make.

✦ Water: One of the easiest things to change is your dog's water supply. Dr. Pitcairn recommends a good-quality water purifier. Author Pat Lazarus strongly recommends buying a water filter to attach to your faucet. She also recommends that if you wish to continue using tap water, let it run for five minutes before you use it. This will help rid the water of eroded heavy metal from your pipes.

+ Veggies and Fruits: These should equal one-third of the daily diet. Use raw or cooked veggies: beans, split peas, lentils, carrots, zucchini, and broccoli are good. Add raw, cut-up fruit occasionally. Organic, unsprayed produce is best.

+ Garlic: Garlic is used widely for animals with various conditions. It can help build the immune system and is a good flea and worm repellent, but it may cause anemia if given for long periods of time. Adding a crushed clove of garlic to your dog's food every day is appropriate.

+ Dairy: Pitcairn recommends raw eggs and cottage cheese. Other possible additions are yogurt and cheddar-type cheese. All provide protein and iron.

+ Grains: Cooked grains should equal one-third of a dog's diet. A few appropriate choices are barley, brown rice, buckwheat, oatmeal, cornmeal, and even crumbled whole wheat bread. These provide carbohydrates.

+ Vitamins: Lazarus would add more vitamin C and E to a general multiple supplement. In fact, many dog specialists recommend additional vitamin C. Vitamin B is also vital for a healthy immune system and can be found in brewer's yeast, another possible daily additive. However, adding arbitrary supplements of vitamins or minerals is generally not recommended without consulting your veterinarian.

+ Oil: Many veterinarians and breeders recommend a tablespoon or two a day of vegetable or canola oil, especially for a dry coat or skin. However, oil may add calories.

+ Meat: Lean, organic meats are best. Turkey, liver, mackerel, chicken, and lamb top most vets' lists. Some recommend raw liver; many recommend raw meat in total. Meat (or some fish) should represent one-third (perhaps a bit more) of the dog's daily diet.

Using Diet to Heal: A Case Study

Throughout this book, I have interspersed university studies with anecdotal evidence with veterinarian's stories. All help me to know how to best treat my own animal companions. Changing a dog's or cat's diet certainly sometimes helps change the course of cancer, no matter how severe the disease may seem.

Lymphoma is one of those cancers in dogs that is hard to treat, and dogs normally may rebound for close to a year, but not much longer. However, there are ways to keep a dog relatively healthy and happy without surgery, X-rays, or chemotherapy.

Dale C. Moss is a classical homeopath who practices in Turners Falls, Massachusetts, and consults on cases involving animals with cancer. His own dog, Ulysses, a black Labrador, came down quite quickly with lymphoma. "Suddenly, Uly's flagging energy and his susceptibility to mange and eye infections made sense; his immune system was deteriorating. I opted not to X-ray him or go for a lymph node biopsy, but instead began to treat him." Of course, he had the homeopathic tools to do so—and a large dog library. "Cancer no longer frightens me since I studied with a wonderful Indian homeopath, Dr. A. U. Ramakrishnan," he wrote. At any rate, Moss came up with the "organ-specific" homeopathic remedies that Ulysses needed. He also changed his diet in accordance with Dr. Pitcairn's advice. "Now Ulysses eats cooked brown rice, finely chopped organic raw vegetables, and chicken, in a 1 to 1 to 1 ratio." This is supplemented by a daily multi-vitamin, flaxseed oil, nutritional yeast, and a teaspoon of vitamin C with each [two a day] meal. "Ulysses' energy is better, his stools have normalized. . . . He even springs up stairs. . . . He'll probably be on this regimen for months, with a rise in potency at some point. But given his response thus far, I trust my faithful friend will be around for years to come."[50]

CATS' NEEDS

Cats have quite different nutritional needs than dogs. They are more truly carnivores than their generally larger friends. They need taurine, an essential amino acid found only in animal tissues. If they do not get this ingredient, cats may have heart problems, go blind, or develop respiratory problems. Blindness was first seen in a taurine-deficient diet when cats were fed only dog food, which does not have to include this ingredient. Cats also need vitamin A, because they can't convert beta-carotene to vitamin A like dogs can. Cats have higher protein requirements than dogs, because they use it as an energy source.[51]

The Association of American Feed Control Officials, which regulates production, analysis, labeling, distribution, and sale of animal feed and livestock remedies, has developed nutrient profiles for four stages of feline life: kittenhood, pregnancy, lactation, and adulthood. Each should include protein, fat, vitamins and minerals, and water. The group does not recommend homemade diets, but rather advises feeding a high-quality commercial cat food that has gone through adequate feeding trials and meets the nutritional criteria established by the organization.[52]

Veterinarians at Tufts University in Boston, Massachusetts, who publish the monthly newsletter *Catnip,* believe that home-cooked meals for cats will, over the long term, lead to vitamin and mineral deficiencies. They warn against a vegetarian diet, because animal tissue is the only natural source of taurine. Dietary supplements will not create nutritional balance either, because they do not contain the correct proportions of nutrients that cats need. "I still see cats coming into the intensive care unit near death because they've been on a vegetarian diet," says Dr. Lisa Freeman, assistant professor and nutritionist at Tufts.

But feeding your cats too much meat is not appropriate either. That diet might be too high in phosphorus and too low in calcium and could lead to various disorders. Dr. Freeman feels that several of the published homemade recipes are not nutritionally balanced. She strongly recommends that if you want to create a nutritionally balanced homemade meal for your cat, you must consult with either a veterinarian or a veterinary nutritionist to find balanced recipes.[53]

A few no-nos for cats are salt and sugar as additives; semimoist food (high in flavoring, artificial colors, preservatives, and so forth); canned tuna; and ham and pork. Canned tuna packaged for humans is worse than that for cats: it contains more mercury. But even canned tuna fish cat food contains high amounts of unsaturated fats and is deficient in vitamin E, an important antioxidant.[54] Here are a few of Anita Frazier's recommendations for treats: "buttered whole wheat toast . . .

a soft-boiled egg . . . an olive . . . cooked meat or poultry . . . a sliver of pizza." As with dogs, *never* feed cats chocolate or cocoa.[55] Fascinatingly, contrary to many of our childhood beliefs, up to 80 percent of animal companions, including cats, cannot tolerate cow's milk, writes Alfred J. Plechner, D.V.M., with Martin Zucker, in *Pets at Risk*. They note that when these pets ingest milk, they may have gassy stomachs, loose stools, vomiting, or diarrhea. Cheese, cottage cheese, and yogurt are much more digestible.[56]

CAT DIET SUGGESTIONS

Cats are a bit fussier than dogs. So what else is new? Here is one diet recommended by Dr. Bodewes: "1 lb. cooked ground beef; $1/4$ cup liver; one cup cooked rice; one tsp. vegetable oil; one tsp. calcium carbonate; and a multi-vitamin/mineral tablet." He suggests that by following rough guidelines, you can substitute protein and carbohydrate sources as desired by you or your finicky feline.[57]

Another diet possibility comes from cat owner Daska Saleeba of Australia. She wanted her cat's story to be told. Her ginger-colored, neutered tabby cat, Snuffy, suffered in early 1999 from what was probably an osteosarcoma and is still alive today at age twelve. He did have a leg amputated. His guardian, Saleeba, feeds this diet to all her cats: "I blend cabbage, celery, parsley, a pet formula of oils, apple cider vinegar, Aloe Vera juice, powdered garlic, soaked psyllium husks, powder wheat grass, coconut, lecithin, and [a powdered food supplement for animals that contains vitamin C, rose hips, kelp, dolomite, and spirulina] which is mixed with kangaroo meat."[58]

Whatever the route you decide to take for your feline's diet—entirely homemade; part homemade, part commercial; or entirely high-quality commercial—remember that cats too need healthy and fresh water every day.

8 Vaccinations

Many veterinarians have become increasingly convinced that a number of vaccines are doing more harm than good for our animal companions. Yes, some remain necessary—even mandated by law, such as rabies. (In the United States rabies vaccinations for cats are currently required in twenty-seven states and the District of Columbia; for dogs, they are required in all states and the District of Columbia.) But not all the traditionally-administered annual boosters now appear to be necessary. And they may be leading to several diseases. Among the conditions associated with vaccines are skin allergies, bladder infections, and even cancer. As W. Jean Dodds, D.V.M., writes, in her article "Changing Vaccine Protocols," "In veterinary medicine, evidence implicating vaccines in triggering immune-mediated and other chronic disorders (vaccinosis) is compelling."[1]

The U.S. veterinary community has been reviewing most vaccine protocols over the last five years and has come to realize that perhaps they have been vaccinating too often. Here's one story of the negative effect of a standard vaccine. Judy Wright's middle-aged golden retriever occasionally had seizures, so she was worried about having him receive the recommended combination booster and rabies vaccine. After she was assured by her veterinarian that revaccination would do no harm, the dog had the shot and, later that day, started having uncontrollable seizures.[2]

When it is time to revaccinate your animal, your veterinarian should consider the pet's age, her lifestyle (indoor or outdoor), her general state of health, the prevalence of the disease in question in the geographic area where you live, whether your animal is pregnant, whether or not you board her, and other factors. Each case is individual and should be considered as such.

One of the more no-holds-barred statements about vaccines is Dr. Richard Pitcairn's warning: "Giving a vaccine to an animal with cancer is like pouring gasoline on a fire."[3] He also advises not vaccinating animal companions who have breast tumors or any other growths or tumors.[4] His overall recommendations regarding vaccines are these: Try to get your veterinarian to give single or simple vaccines rather than complex vaccines. Young animals can tolerate a reduced vaccination schedule, but vaccinating is not advised before sixteen weeks of age. And annual boosters—which don't have "much justification"—should be avoided, even though they have long been popular. Pitcairn goes so far as to advise against "any further vaccinations after the initial series, as they are not necessary." He adds that the latest official medical opinion is that annual boosters are neither required nor effective, although not all veterinarians will agree with or even know this fact.[5]

W. Jean Dodds, D.V.M., one of the world's experts in canine vaccine reactions and owner of Hemopet in Santa Monica, California, which provides titering services for both dogs and cats, says, "Recent vaccinations with single or combination modified live virus (MLV) vaccines are increasingly recognised contributors to immune-mediated blood diseases, bone marrow failure, and organ dysfunction." She lists thyroid disease, Addison's disease, diabetes, leukemia, and lymphoma as among the diseases that can be triggered by these vaccines.[6]

Christina Chambreau, D.V.M., incorporates homeopathic and holistic therapies into her veterinary practice. She writes, "Holistic veterinarians are finding that vaccines are causing great harm to our animals (and ourselves). . . . Conventional veterinarians are also reporting health problems due to vaccinations. . . . Reports include: immunological disorders; adverse vaccine reactions; increased sensitivity to pollen antigens after vaccination."

In answer to the question "Can my animals really be safe and healthy without vaccinations?" Dr. Chambreau responds vehemently "Yes!" She cites dog trainers and writers Wendy and Jack Volhard, who have studied dog kennels in Germany. They observed more than two hundred dogs who are given only a distemper vaccine and parvovirus vaccines at ten weeks and then at one year and are occasionally given rabies shots, when needed. These dogs have litters, show at ten years of age, and live to be sixteen or so. "In the States, many shepherds are dying by the age of 10," Chambreau explains. "Other breeders have found that stopping vaccination has made their line much healthier, and usually immune (through good health) to the infectious agents that can cause disease. Not always, of course. Some dogs or cats are very susceptible to disease and will become infected and may die. Most survive epidemics with mild disease, if treated holistically."[7]

It should be noted that veterinarians derive a sizable amount of income from administering vaccines. "Many practices generate 15% to 25% of their gross incomes from vaccination visits," writes Gary D. Norsworthy, D.V.M. "This income is supplemented by fees for additional services generated by the vaccination visit (e.g., dental procedures). . . . The immediate result of extended vaccination intervals will be the loss of this relatively easily generated income. Some veterinary practices may not be able to survive financially. Those operating on close profit margins and depending heavily on vaccination income will be the first fatalities."[8]

In news first published in the American Animal Hospital Association's *NEWStat,* two animal-related bills were defeated and expired that "would have required veterinarians to disclose vaccine risks to clients." The bills were introduced in Maine and Nevada. Both were defeated in April 2005. This would have been the first such regulation in the country, although Veterinary Medical Association members say that such protection for their clients already exists in the Veterinary Practice Act.[9]

VACCINE-INDUCED FELINE SARCOMAS

I am not advocating giving up all vaccines for your animals; each case is different, and you should obtain information and guidance from a trusted (and up-to-date) animal care practitioner. However, you should be especially careful and prepared regarding one type of vaccination that has, over the past fifteen years, actually produced malignant tumors or sarcomas in cats. Our cat Puck died of this virulent cancer, which is caused by killed-virus leukemia and rabies vaccines that are traditionally administered between the shoulder blades. Let me describe this disease, the vaccines that can cause it, and how you might avoid it for your feline companions.

About twenty-two million cats received vaccinations in 1991. Those numbers are undoubtedly higher today. In surveys conducted in 1992 estimates were that between twenty-two hundred and twenty-two thousand cats per year were developing aggressive fibrosarcomas after receiving those vaccinations,[10] at an average of eight years of age. The risk has been climbing in the past five to ten years, at least in the United States. Every veterinarian I have talked to in the past two years has seen at least one cat with this condition. Most animals, unfortunately, do not survive long.

Denise Kessler, D.V.M., in Charlotte, Vermont, has seen three cats in four and a half years with vaccine-induced sarcomas. Of the three, the cat who lived the longest was treated by surgery, two cycles of chemotherapy, and herbal treatments (she uses Essiac and milk thistle for many cat cases). This middle-aged cat has survived for three years now, certainly a success story for this type of cancer. The other two cats were treated with surgery alone.

George Glanzberg, V.M.D., of North Bennington, Vermont, practices both conventional and homeopathic medicine. He has seen no vaccine-related sarcomas in his own patients, in part because he uses very little leukemia vaccine in his practice. However, he notes, "Several cases have come to us after surgery in other offices which were presumed to be FeLV vaccine associated. All have been on dorsal neck or somewhat distal to dorsal neck. Treatment has been homeopathic and survival time has been less than two years in all cases." He concludes, "But they were advanced at the beginning of our therapy."[11]

Some statistics put the risk of this sarcoma at between one in a thousand and one in ten thousand, but those numbers are probably changing monthly. Before 1985 feline fibrosarcoma was rare (as it still is in countries where animals are rarely vaccinated). That date marks the introduction of killed-virus rabies and leukemia vaccines. Following this, rabies vaccinations became mandatory for cats in many states.

Dr. Norsworthy explains: "In the mid- to late 1980s, a basic change occurred in the vaccine manufacturing process. By order of the U.S.

Department of Agriculture, manufacturers shifted most of their vaccines from modified live virus to killed products. To maximize the immune response to these killed antigens, the manufacturers incorporated aluminum into the adjuvants." Around 1991 veterinarians began to notice a higher number of sarcomas in the sites where vaccines were injected.[12] Norsworthy continues, "The addition of aluminum was considered a likely cause of the sarcomas." He points to particles of aluminum found within the tumor cells and in "macrophages several centimeters from the tumor" as additional evidence of their culpability.

Further, a columnist for *CATS Magazine* has noted, "Of special interest to the medical community is the frequency with which aluminum appears in these affected tissues. . . . Other metals have also been found to induce sarcoma formation in certain conditions. They include arsenic, chromium and nickel. Metallic implants have even been associated with osteosarcomas."[13]

Still, Dr. Norsworthy admits that aluminum is only a *likely* factor. "We still don't know exactly what causes these tumors."[14] Amy Marder, V.M.D., agrees that the veterinary community does not yet understand why some vaccines promote cancer while others don't. "One theory is that it's caused by certain additives in the solution," she notes. "Those additives might cause inflammation, which can sometimes bring on a malignant reaction in normal cells. Specifically, some scientists speculate, the aluminum in some formulas may be at the root of the problem. Others believe that the tumors develop because the vaccines deliver such a high concentration of virus to such a small area." She recommends making sure your veterinarian is avoiding aluminum in vaccine formulas, along with asking him or her to use a modified live-virus form of vaccine.[15]

In a study performed by Dr. D. W. Macy and Dr. P. J. Bergman, thirty-six cats received rabies and feline leukemia vaccines. "Within three weeks, 80% to 100% of cats had local reactions to rabies vaccination, depending on the brand used and whether or not that brand contained aluminum. Feline leukemia vaccine containing aluminum produced the highest number of reactions and vaccine with no adjuvant at all produced no reactions." Although there were twice as many reactions to the rabies vaccines as to the leukemia, other studies have found fewer sarcomas at the rabies vaccination site than at the leukemia site.[16]

Philip H. Kass, D.V.M., found that FeLV vaccines have a slightly greater potential for causing these sarcomas than rabies vaccines, although the latter is not without its implications. He adds, "The number of cats whose sarcomas are linked to FeLV and rabies vaccines, respectively, is a function not only of the tumorigenic potential of the vaccines, but also of how often the vaccines are used." He follows with the example of Hawaii—where the rabies vaccine is not given, thus "presumably all vaccine-associated sarcomas are caused by the FeLV vaccine."[17]

Because of a rising concern about this problem, the Vaccine-Associated Feline Sarcoma Task Force, a coalition of concerned national veterinary organizations that wish to resolve this dilemma, formed in 1996. The task force consists of representatives from the American Veterinary Medical Association, the American Animal Hospital Association, the American Association of Feline Practitioners, and the Veterinary Cancer Society, along with other veterinary researchers and government and animal care representatives. They devote human and financial resources to examine the causes and most effective treatment of sarcomas. As of 2003, these were their recommendations: Always look at a number of issues when deciding to vaccinate your cats. These include "risk of exposure to the disease-causing organism . . . the consequence of infection; the risk an infected cat poses to human health; the protective ability of the vaccine; the frequency or severity of reactions the vaccine produces; the age and health status of your cat; and vaccine reactions your cat may have experienced in the past."[18]

The task force had the following recommendations regarding these common feline vaccines: feline panleukopenia virus vaccine (feline distemper) (highly recommended for all cats by the task force); feline calicivirus/herpesvirus vaccine (highly recommended by the task force); rabies virus vaccine (apparently rabies poses a serious threat to cats of today and rabies shots for cats are now required in many states); feline leukemia virus (this vaccine is recommended for "all cats at risk of exposure to the virus," indoor cats are obviously at less risk).

As is true for dogs now, vaccination with a "triennially-approved rabies vaccine every three years" is now considered sufficient. Research points to evidence that the panlekopenia/rhinotracheitis/ calicivirus vaccines generally last for several years, but many veterinarians now recommend these be given every three years as well.

The task force does not believe that vaccines are inherently "dangerous," but warns that "there is a small chance that reactions may develop as a result of vaccination." The task force recommends always consulting your veterinarian if your cat experiences any kind of adverse reaction to a vaccine.[19]

According to Tom Elston, D.V.M., a member of the Feline Sarcoma Task Force, and owner of T.H.E. Cat Hospital in Irvine, California, hard, cold statistics on feline-induced fibrosarcomas and the damage they cause are difficult to come by. "Veterinary medicine keeps poor records on these kinds of things."[20] However, he did discuss the latest study, published in 2002 in *The Journal of the American Veterinary Association*. "No one knows the exact number for sure. But one epidemiological study looked at 30,000 vaccines given to 15,000 cats—one fibrosarcoma developed. However, previous studies had shown that one in 10,000 and even one in 1,000 cats developed this fibrosarcoma." The Task Force is in the process of dissolving after working together for ten years, he explained, because "We have done some good research, we started answering some questions, and the AVMA thought we had done enough and wasn't backing us any longer."

One change that may have helped the cats has been a change in the location of the administration of some shots. Dr. Elston even has a few long-time survivors of this feline fibrosarcoma: "If we do it on the leg, we can amputate if necessary." And he added that more good news for animal companions is that future guidelines (beyond the latest listed here) for vaccines may spread some out even longer than the current guidelines call for. Some vaccines may last a lifetime, others as long as six years.[21]

Dr. Dodds pointed out an amazing new study to me. The study was done on dogs in Italy between seven months and eleven years old. While in cats the fibrosarcoma is the second most prevalent skin tumor, in dogs it is quite rare. However, in this study, which was published in the *Journal of Veterinary Medicine* in 2003, "fifteen fibrosarcomas, surgically excised from presumed sites of injection in dogs, and 10 canine fibrosarcomas excised from sites not used for injection were histologically and immunohistochemically compared with 20 feline post-vaccine fibrosarcomas." The researchers found similarities between the two species, "suggesting the possibility of the development of post-injection sarcomas not only in cats, but also in dogs."[22]

CANINE VACCINES

The protocol for canine vaccines has also changed in the last five years, in favor of giving fewer vaccines. This is exceedingly good news. According to the American Animal Hospital Association (AAHA) Canine Vaccine Task Force's 2003 Canine Vaccine Guidelines, "Current knowledge supports the statement that no vaccine is always safe, no vaccine is always protective, and no vaccine is always indicated."[23]

Canine distemper virus, CPV (canine parvovirus), canine adenovirus-2, and rabies virus are considered the "core" vaccines. The first three (distemper, CPV, and adenovirus-2) should be administered to all puppies and to dogs "with an unknown vaccination history." After that "revaccination every three years is considered protective." The rabies virus is slightly different. All puppies and dogs with unknown histories should have the initial shot and then a booster 12 months after. Thereafter, they should receive these shots "as required by local, state, or provincial law." However, "The minimum DOI (duration of immunity) for killed rabies vaccine based on challenge studies is 3 years; based on antibody titers, it is considered to be up to 7 years." Although this shot's effects can last quite a long time, veterinarians advocate abiding by the laws.

This canine task force also recommends looking at the animal's environment, age, breed, health status, and lifestyle before vaccinating. Under the environmental factors to consider, they conclude, "Exposure to trauma (automobiles, fights, etc.), weather, water, toxins, sunlight, as well as internal and external parasites should be assessed during annual health-care visits in order to define risk factors and appropriate preventive measures." Dogs that stay in kennels, or visit grooming salons, dog parks, doggy daycare, or tick-infested areas are at higher risk from certain infections than those who do not do these things. (We never take our dog to areas known to have high tick populations because we don't want to have to vaccinate against ticks.)

Finally, the AAHA Canine Vaccine Task Force humbly explains "The burgeoning knowledge in the fields of vaccinology and immunology

. . . have placed the traditional approach to vaccine use in doubt and engaged our profession in a long overdue debate. . . . One size simply does not fit all. Not all vaccines are indicated in all animals and no vaccine should be given without a thorough knowledge of the risks of acquiring the disease, the potential for adverse reactions to vaccination, and the health of the animal in question."[24]

ALTERNATIVES TO VACCINATION

Nosodes

One alternative to many vaccines is nosodes. These are homeopathic preparations made from a diseased animal's tissues; they contain not only the disease organism but also the animal's response to the organism. Many veterinarians and animal guardians have been using nosodes on an ongoing basis, although they are somewhat controversial. Dr. Chambreau says, "Some are using nosodes for each disease, and others are using a combination of all the diseases." However, she also notes, "This is still operating from a fear of getting something, rather than a proactive stance of 'let's become very healthy so that even if we are exposed to a communicable disease, we will not get that ill.'"[25]

Catherine O'Driscoll of England, author of *Who Killed the Darling Buds of May,* a recent book about the dangers of vaccines for animals, says that existing research and experience show nosodes to be at least as protective as vaccines. "Whereas the medical and veterinary 'professions' receive huge sums of money from international multi-billion dollar pharmaceutical conglomerates, please note that homeopaths do not. Rather, vets who trust the less expensive homeopathic alternative suffer serious financial loss by refusing to sell highly lucrative annual boosters." Dog lovers, in particular, are beginning to choose nosodes as an alternative to vaccines. Some have used nosodes for twenty years and have never had a resultant health problem.[26]

Still, Jane Bicks, D.V.M., a veterinarian for approximately twenty years who now uses a holistic approach to animal care, is not certain about nosodes. "Experts don't seem to agree upon their efficacy. I for one am afraid to leave a cat without the protection of a true vaccine, because nursing a cat with one of these diseases back to health is very difficult, if possible at all. Rabies has no cure! I am confident that the medical community will come up with a new vaccinations regime that will be safe and effective. In the meanwhile, discuss your concerns with your family veterinarian," she writes.[27]

Nosodes are not yet used widely. In an extensive, although not exhaustive, search of my home state of Vermont, for example, I did not find any veterinarians who used them, even among those with a holistic bent. However, perhaps a search of the AltVetMed Web site (www.altvetmed.org) would produce the name of a veterinarian in your area who is already using this therapy. You can also search by state, country, modality, and type of practice on the American Holistic Veterinary Medical Association Web site (www.ahvma.org). (See the resources at the end of this book for additional contact information.)

Titering

Several holistic-minded veterinarians are now taking advantage of a process called titering, in which blood samples are drawn and then laboratory-tested to determine the animal's immunity levels. Only if the animal really needs a certain vaccine is it administered. One of the most famous titering centers is Hemopet, a nonprofit animal blood bank in California run by Jean Dodds, D.V.M.

Although Hemopet began in 1990, Dodds has been working on the vaccination issue for more than three decades. Her lab began titering more than ten years ago. Explains Dr. Dodds, "I helped our lab (Antech Diagnostics) set up the new IFA [immunofluorescent assay] method which we validated and published in our national veterinary journal in 2000. This is still the largest vaccine titer study published to date."[28]

For dogs, the lab titers for distemper, parvovirus, occasionally rabies ("for proven severe reactors to earlier vaccinations"), hepatitis, parainfluenza, leptospirosis, coronavirus, and Lyme disease. For cats, it performs titering for panleukopenia (mostly), calicivirus, herpes virus, and leukemia virus. Dodds began offering this service for pets "because we overvaccinate. The frequency of adverse reactions is unacceptable." Titering "avoids unnecessary risks and the cost of vaccines," she explains. People from all over North America and other countries send in blood samples for testing by Dr. Dodds. Although hers was one of the first labs to administer titering, many other laboratories now offer the service as well, including those at most veterinary teaching hospitals. Ask your vet if titering is offered at any of the labs in your area or any of those that he or she uses regularly. If your vet does not offer the possibility of titer testing, agrees Dodds, "The well-informed dog and cat pet caregiver definitely SHOULD request this type of titer testing in lieu of booster vaccination, except for rabies vaccine."[29]

Dr. Dodds notes a study performed in the 1990s of dogs vaccinated between nine and fifty-five months previously. Results indicated that 73 percent of the 122 dogs had protective canine parvovirus (CPV) titers, and 79 percent of 117 dogs were adequately protected against canine distemper virus. The study's authors concluded that "annual revaccination should be maintained, because less than 90% of those vaccinated reached their criteria for protective titers."

However, Dr. Dodds and Lisa Twark, D.V.M., came to quite a different conclusion. They write, "Our study evaluated 1441 dogs for CPV antibody titer and 1379 dogs for CDV antibody titer. Of these, 95% were judged to have adequate CPV titers, and nearly all (98%) had adequate CDV titers." The majority of the dogs who participated in the study had been vaccinated one or two years prior to the study. On the basis of this data, the two veterinarians concluded that "annual revaccination is unnecessary."[30]

Dr. Dodds believes the new vaccination protocol of every three years is a "step in the right direction." But she and other veterinarians prefer a "case-by-case approach. This would mean giving appropriately spaced puppy or kitten vaccines (2 or 3 doses only, starting at 8–10 weeks), another booster at one year, and then titers thereafter, except for rabies, as required by law."[31]

Thuja

If you decide that you cannot risk not giving your animals the vaccines still recommended by your veterinarian, you might consider asking if the animal could also be given thuja. This homeopathic remedy from the North American white cedar tree is used by many holistically inclined veterinarians as an antidote for vaccines and the chronic conditions resulting from them. Dr. Goldstein notes that "I keep a little squirt bottle of thuja in the refrigerator at the clinic. When I give a pet a vaccine (one of the very few he'll get from me!), I give him a squirt in the mouth; usually I'll give him another squirt to two when I next see him."[32]

Dr. Richard Pitcairn feels that thuja is one of the most important remedies for vaccine-related illnesses. In many cases the progress of his patients was dependent on the use of thuja. He says that it is not necessarily the final remedy, but "it seemed to be a necessary prescription. It is as if vaccinations have the ability to block response to a constitutional remedy, an obstacle that must be dealt with before cure can be underway. Sometimes, when the picture is muddled, perhaps because of prior treatment with allopathic drugs, Thuja can bring clarity into the situation."[33]

Dr. Pitcairn continues, "I believe that the attitudes and feelings people now have about vaccinations are the same ones people used to have about bleedings. The prominent doctors, all the most important authorities, agreed they [the bleedings] were absolutely beneficial. Anyone who dared to question that assumption was ridiculed. Now we look back on that practice with amazement. . . . I trust we will be doing the same thing someday when we look back at the practice of vaccination."[34]

9 The Role of Emotions

Emotions play heavily in disease—in both its formation and its treatment. This is true for animals' ailments as well as those of humans. In an animal's illness emotions at play are threefold: those of the animal; those of her human companion; and those of the presiding veterinarian in his or her relationship with both the animal and the owner.

Most people today realize that animals feel emotions. They are similar to us in many ways. Gary Kowalski, a Unitarian Universalist minister and author of *The Souls of Animals* and *Goodbye Friend: Healing Wisdom for Anyone Who Has Ever Lost a Pet,* addresses animals' emotions in his two books. In chapter 1 of *The Souls of Animals* he wonders what it means for an animal to be spiritually evolved: "It means many things: the development of a moral sense, the appreciation of beauty, the capacity for creativity, and the awareness of one's self within a larger universe as well as a sense of mystery and wonder about it all."[1]

In his chapter "The Eyes of Hope," in which he tackles the issue of animals' self-consciousness, he advises readers to look deeply into another animal's eyes, to have an "interspecies meditation." He writes, "This is a creature who is alive and has desires like you. It walks the same ground and breathes the same air. It feels pain and enjoys its senses . . . as you do. And in this we are all kin."[2]

In the final chapter of *The Souls of Animals,* Kowalski once again addresses the question of animals having souls. He describes their emotional lives as "nuanced with moods that range from grief and sadness to gaiety and glee." He calls animals "our peers and fellow travelers. Like us, they have their own likes and dislikes, fears and fixations. . . . Animals not only have biologies; they also have biographies"[3] (an idea for which he credits Tom Regan, professor of religion and philosophy at North Carolina State University).

In her moving autobiographical book *Reason for Hope,* Jane Goodall, famous for her studies of chimpanzees, writes about collecting scientific data and feeling empathy with her subjects. "In order to collect good, scientific data, one is told, it is necessary to be coldly objective," she begins. "You record accurately what you see and, above all, you do not permit yourself to have any empathy with your subjects. Fortunately I did not know that during the early months at Gombe. A great deal of my understanding of these intelligent beings was built up just *because* I felt such empathy with them. Once you know *why* something happens, you can test your interpretation as rigorously as you like. There are still scientists around nowadays who will raise supercilious eyebrows if you talk of empathy with animals, but attitudes are beginning to soften."[4]

THE HUMAN-ANIMAL BOND

Not only do animals have emotions, but when they live with us they seem to pick up on our human emotions—and even sometimes on our illnesses. We know that if we are sick or feel discouraged, our animal companions (dogs in particular) want to be at our side to comfort us. When I had the flu this past fall, my dog and one of my cats spent the whole day sleeping by my side in bed. They are normally much more active during the day. It is a known fact that humans and animals can affect each other's pulse and heart rates, writes Myrna M. Milani, D.V.M., in *The Art of Veterinary Practice: A Guide to Client Communication.*[5]

Dr. Milani adds that it is not unreasonable to also suggest that animal companions can become upset when they see their guardians distressed. She notes that an animal who maintains a close relationship with her human will probably share the same lifestyle and may, in some cases, eat the same high-salt, high-fat foods or follow other "unhealthy practices that may undermine the animal's health." Because an animal companion is smaller and lives a shorter time, related health problems will show up earlier in a dog or cat.[6]

Whereas the results of many human-animal studies showing that animals make us feel better have been widely available for decades, studies now show that we, in turn, can make animals feel better. In her book Milani mentions several studies that reveal that animals who are treated well feel better. For instance, a study of rabbit diets was performed at the Ohio State University College of Medicine by Frederick Cornhill. In it the animals' blood cholesterol levels were tested after a specific feeding period. Cornhill discovered that some rabbits' cholesterol levels were 50 percent lower than the others. The difference was that the healthier animals had been especially well cared for by a technician, who held and stroked as well as fed them every day. Milani explains, "Other work offers compelling evidence that nothing more or less than our concerned presence and touch can make animals feel better, too."[7]

Dr. Milani told me that it is reasonable to assume mood and stress can affect a nonhuman animal as they do a human. She points to studies that show an animal's position in its social structure can affect its levels of substances such as cortisol and testosterone. "Because cortisol plays such a critical role in the immune response, it seems reasonable to me that, for example, a more subordinate animal inadvertently thrust into a leadership position in the human-canine pack by an unknowledgeable owner, or a naturally more submissive solitary cat forced to live in a confined space with other cats could wind up with a double whap of cortisol during periods of stress. Do that long enough and it's also conceivable that the immune response would break down, which, if turned on the animal's own cells, could set it up for cancer as well as other immune-related problems." Dr. Milani believes that addressing these issues is a necessary first step for practicing integrated body-mind medicine in both nonhuman and human animals.[8]

Donna Raditic, D.V.M., a veterinarian who practices conventional medicine and also is a certified acupuncturist and a specialist in nutrition, believes that animal companions' jobs are to take on our grief, anger, and unresolved issues. This is what a domestic animal's purpose is, she believes. She says, "This is meant to tell us, we should be happier. . . . And through our happiness, they will stay healthier." Of course, animals also have their own emotional lives, but their mental state is affected by the humans with whom they live. "They would be perfect if we weren't there. Their job is to receive all our fears, our insecurities, willingly."[9]

Dr. Raditic is not alone in this opinion. One animal lover and provider put it this way: Molly Sheehan of Green Hope Farm, which produces and markets Flower Essences says, "Animals pick up and carry the stress of people they live with and even people they just run into. This is their job description as members of the Elemental kingdom. Their job description is, in part, to absorb our negativity and help us find balance." Sheehan doesn't just sell products to animal lovers; she is a big-time animal fan too: she lives with two golden retrievers, one cat, and twenty fish and has had chickens. "We have grown more appreciative, some would say nutty, over our animals as our work with the Essences continues. Animals are SUCH discerning clients and use Essences with such skill and grace!"[10]

Another veterinarian, Darren Hawks, D.V.M., puts it this way: "In some cases, pets may come in to their owner's lives with the 'soul purpose' of living out the role of a sick pet to enable both the pet and its owner to learn soul lessons (grief, love, etc.). At times the pet-owner bond is based on the pet being sick so the owner can act as a caretaker. In such cases, both the pet and the owner must be part of the healing if real progress is to be made."[11]

Betsy Adams of Ann Arbor, Michigan, would agree. She has been working with animals for twenty-five years. Her holistic healing, behavior counseling, and other animal services practice is called the Animal/Human Energy Bond. When she began her work with creatures and "their humans," she "observed in each animal client the obvious compassionate manner in which animals 'took on' or 'down-loaded' their humans' issues." She feels that these animals were helping their people get back on track with their work on this earth. "The animals were on a parallel path with their human," she writes. "They were tracking the human and mirroring back what the human was really doing in this life here—not what we desire, not what we want, but the true intention behind all our choices." Animals take on our angers, depressions, and fears, but they do not complain, even though they sometimes get sick. "They are, above all, totally compassionate where their humans are concerned."

Adams feels strongly that animals "need a vacation, and so do we, from the attitude and misconception that we are victims, that we have no power. We are not victims, and we do have power! That is why the animals have never given up on us."[12]

As I was revising this book and adding new information, a friend rented the film, *Best in Show,* about dog shows and dog-human relationships. One relationship in this film certainly points out how our moods and personalities can affect the animals with whom we live. A young yuppie couple lived with a beautiful Weimeraner, who they were preparing for a prestigious show. The dog would become agitated when he saw the couple having sex, and the couple often argued and became quite hysterical. At the show, they somehow lost the dog's favorite chewy toy and began screaming and running around frantically, just before the dog was due to compete. When it was the right class for their dog, they took him out to the runway, and he almost immediately barked at and lunged toward the judge! Wouldn't any of us react in some uncharacteristic way, considering all the built-up stress and emotion?[13]

DURING CANCER THERAPY

It can sometimes be difficult to cope when your pet is suffering, will not eat, cannot jump up on the bed, or does not want to go for a walk. As Samantha Mooney writes in *A Snowflake in My Hand,* about the Animal Medical Center in New York, where she worked with cats with cancer: "When a pet is sick, there is an ever-present weight that burdens us throughout the day. Sometimes we are not even consciously aware of it until it is lifted, like a persistent headache that becomes a part of our normal sensations."[14] Yet no matter how hard it is, we must maintain our good relationship with our sick animal companions, and try to remain hopeful and optimistic for their future.

Dr. Raditic makes a case for maintaining a strong human-animal bond during cancer therapy, no matter what that therapy is. She believes that veterinarians often need to play a role in helping guardians come to terms with the creature's disease. "I spend a great deal of time educating owners about the pet's emotions regarding their disease and eventual death. I try to identify the owner's and his pet's priorities and work very hard to maintain them both as long as possible. I believe it is important to strive for quality life, *not* quantity . . . that is what most of our animal friends want," she says. Raditic believes that animals do not fear death like we humans do. "I find this [understanding] very rewarding, spiritual, and comforting. It has given me a basis for dealing with our mortality and perhaps some insight into the meaning of life." In her practice it is especially gratifying to become a part of the relationship between a human and his or her animal companion. "That is a very special place indeed," she adds.[15]

Dr. Milani believes that all clinicians and veterinarians should make an assessment of the guardians' relationships to the animals, their expectations for treatment, and the implication that those expectations can play a critical role in successful treatment of any serious condition. She believes veterinarians should begin to collect that information during the first appointment.[16] Although in my experience this does not generally happen, certainly this mirrors what Vermont homeopathic veterinarian George Glanzberg told me he does when first seeing an animal (see chapter 14, Homeopathy and Naturopathy).

Jerrold Tannenbaum, professor of veterinary ethics and law at the University of California Davis School of Veterinary Medicine, recently spoke about the ethics of veterinary medicine. "In many respects, veterinary medical ethics is more difficult than human medical ethics. Physicians serve the interests of their patients. But from the very beginning, veterinarians have had two masters. Animals are their patients; clients or owners pay the bill.

"What makes veterinary ethics sometimes so difficult and so intriguing is that the interests of the patient can conflict with the interests of the client. Veterinarians are sometimes caught in the middle, wanting to serve both."[17]

EMOTIONAL STRESS

In his book *Earl Mindell's Nutrition and Health for Dogs,* the author notes that emotional stress can affect a dog's immune system. "Most dogs are very sensitive to their owner's emotions," he writes, pointing to a recurring connection between bone cancer in dogs and stress found by researcher Dr. Beverly Cappel-King. In most of the cases of bone cancer she has treated, she finds there has been recent stress in the living situation—such as divorce or illness. One example was Hilda, a four-year-old Doberman. Hilda and her guardian were inseparable. The guardian worked only part time away from the home. When Hilda's guardian got a second job, though, it took just three months until the dog began limping on her left front leg and was diagnosed with bone cancer. The guardian immediately quit her second job and made Hilda "the center of her life." Dr. Cappel-King gave Hilda antioxidants, herbs, vitamins, and other alternative treatments to build up her immune system. Six months later, with no surgery, X-rays showed Hilda's bone to be free of cancer. Three and a half years later the dog was still cancer-free. Cappel-King attributed the recovery more to the guardian's positive, loving attitude than to her remedies.

This is how stress can hurt your animals: It increases the production of adrenaline, which can then suppress and shrink the thymus gland. Because this gland produces many white blood cells, stress can lead to a deficiency of these cells and suppression of the immune system—making your animal more susceptible to disease. Stress has also been known to trigger autoimmune diseases such as arthritis and hemolytic anemia in dogs. For dogs that are highly and frequently stressed, Earl Mindell recommends naturally calming remedies such as B-complex vitamins, magnesium, homeopathic remedies, valerian, and kava.[18]

In cats, especially, stress is known to play a large role in illness. According to animal writer Anita Frazier, cats have a lower stress threshold than humans. Prolonged stress can "wear on their nerves and eventually leaves them vulnerable to disease." Stress can also activate a latent disease or pathological condition already in the body.[19]

A few stressors for cats include: surprises; loud noises; the guardian's unhappiness or distress; environmental changes; new visitors; being left alone; being caged; X-rays, anesthesia, or medications; preservatives in foods, supplements, or hairball remedies; obesity; pain; strong smells; trauma or fright; and so on. At the very least, Frazier recommends being as thoughtful as possible, feeding a nutritious diet, and keeping stress to a minimum.[20]

HOPE AND OPTIMISM

We have all heard about the power of faith, prayer, and positive thinking in human cancer patients' recoveries. This philosophy is not news. But this line of thinking also can apply to the comfort, remission, or recovery of animal cancer patients.

Kathleen Griffin, N.D., a naturopathic healer of animals in Australia, recently saw both a dog with stomach cancer and a cat with osteosarcoma. "The animal guardians of both cases refused to focus on the disease but focused rather on wellness. I believe this is the key to cancer treatment. The most powerful treatment for cancer, I therefore believe, is positive thought therapy. There is a well-known saying: 'that which we focus on, we get more of.' "[21] She believes that the reason so many people and animals die "needlessly" from cancer each year is in part because there's so much fear about the disease. "If we can regard cancer as just another symptom of incorrect living and work about rebalancing the mind, body and spirit in a natural way," there will be less cancer.

In a professional course Griffin offers on the philosophy of natural care (it is part of a two-year Diploma of Natural Animal Care course, which provides training in a variety of modalities for natural animal therapists), she tells her students: "Remember, your thoughts and the thoughts of others are all powerful. Always offer hope to others. You can explain to an animal's carer [caregiver] that you cannot predict the destiny of an animal's soul and that all things are possible; you can also explain that whatever the outcome, it will be in keeping with divine providence, but always give hope because without hope there cannot be a positive outcome!"[22]

In the past decade and a half the work of Larry Dossey, M.D., has addressed some similar issues. He is most famous, perhaps, for his strong ideas on the power of prayer in healing. He is the author of *Prayer Is Good Medicine* and other books, and executive editor of *Alternative Therapies in Health and Medicine*. Dr. Dossey recently spoke at length about the power of prayer and positive thinking, referring to at least 150 studies that demonstrate statistically that distant intercessory prayer (prayer at a distance on behalf of someone other than yourself) does have effects. Even though it is difficult to explain exactly how this works in formal scientific lingo, Dossey says, "I think we have to say that there are simply things that consciousness can mediate or consciousness can do that the brain or the body are incapable of. This is a way of saying that the mind is more than the brain and the body." Although he would like it if more hard evidence existed about this relationship, he admits such proof may be a long time coming.

Dr. Dossey understands that the "more radical a therapy is, the more fear it stirs up in doctors," because of this lack of clear evidence. Even though he admits that many types of alternative healing, including healing on the body-mind-spirit level, have always been popular and effective in many countries and cultures besides the United States, in this country "we've been willing to say, particularly within medicine, that if you can't measure it and define it and subdivide it, it doesn't exist." Regardless of these attitudes, which he clearly does not share, Dossey knows that when people pray, good things happen. "Prayer has a powerful, healthful effect on the body."[23] Certainly, praying calmly for your animal companion's well-being during painful times cannot hurt her recovery and treatment. Animals know when you are upset, and generally react well to calmness.

Whether we pray or not, we can provide our animals with psychological support. Richard Pitcairn, D.V.M., notes that a guardian's emotions and expectations can sometimes influence an animal companion's health status. A calm, positive response to an animal's symptoms can relax and reassure the animal, which in turn strengthens the creature's immune response. Over the years Dr. Pitcairn has repeatedly observed that the animals most likely to recover from chronic and difficult illnesses are those whose guardians remain calm and positive. He does, however, advise not to worry unduly over whether your emotional state has affected your animal's health. That will do no one any good. Instead, he advises remaining as comfortable, calm, and self-assured as possible for the good of your animal and for the good of the treatment procedures.[24]

Anna Guitton, D.V.M., of Villars en Pons, France, agrees: "The vibration around a cancer (or any seriously ill) patient is important. It affects, to a great extent, the amount of commitment and the decisions that can be made in the running (management) of the treatment."[25]

Carolyn Ashton, a natural therapy veterinarian in Australia, advocates getting the entire family involved when your animal has a serious disease such as cancer, "especially children, adolescents, or anybody that has a closer relationship with the animal. It is hard to focus on healing when you are all feeling desolated by the potential of your pet's death." She also advocates a new attitude toward the word *healing:* "Too often we associate the word *healing* with survival. Many times I see healing happen, even when the animal dies. I know this idea is receiving focus amongst the human health field, and it is no less appropriate for animals. After all, their situations greatly mirror ours."[26]

Finally, it is important for the veterinarian to remain optimistic. George Glanzberg, V.M.D., tells me, "I really don't know which animal will get well and which one will not, so I don't give up even in the face of severest illness. It is very important for me to remain optimistic when I am working, even when I have to make the family aware that a negative outcome might occur."[27]

COPING WITH DEATH

The way that the human copes with the process and with the loss of a beloved animal companion can also affect the kind of death the animal has. A recent example comes to mind. My friend Rita Reynolds, publisher and editor of *laJoie,* a journal that celebrates all beings, in Batesville, Virginia, lost a sweet ten-year-old white mixed-breed terrier named Oliver to bladder cancer after a tough three-month battle. She writes, "Cancer is a monster, yet I also came to the realization that by hating the cancer, I was hating his cells, thus the very blocks he was made of. So, I gave up the anger and hatred and settled for blessing and love. In the end I think it made a difference. . . . I guess I could say that Oliver is fine now, having a blast rushing around in the spirit world, finally free of pain and suffering. He certainly deserves it."[28]

Because she generally houses approximately twenty-five dogs and cats at a time, often dropped off at her home, it is not unusual for Reynolds to lose creatures to cancer. She has lost dogs, cats, and a duck to the disease. Each time becomes a bit harder, stoic and spiritual though Reynolds may remain. Not surprisingly, she has just written a book about conscious-dying work with animals, *Blessing the Bridge: What Animals Teach Us about Death, Dying, and Beyond.*

PHASES OF ACCEPTANCE

Dr. Milani notes that the phases that humans experience as they come to grips with terminal conditions in animals mirror the five-stage process physician Elisabeth Kübler-Ross described for dying humans and their loved ones in her seminal book, *On Death and Dying*. These are denial, anger, bargaining, depression, and acceptance. This latter stage is what Reynolds expresses so eloquently.

Dr. Milani believes that "owners coping with the death of an animal go through the same five-step process that attended the acceptance of its dying condition." Denial is often short lived because it is quite difficult to perpetuate. She believes that client anger may create negative results for the veterinarian. Sometimes clients lash out at the staff and faculty of a teaching hospital or at the doctor who treated their dog or cat in her last days. Milani definitely recommends that a clinician, at the end of the entire process, make some comment recognizing a positive aspect of the grieving client's relationship with the animal. An "unembarrassed hug" is appropriate at these times, too. Milani believes that such interactions can do much to speed the transition from the animal guardian's depression to their final acceptance of death—and to their ability to move on.[29] For more on coping with an animal companion's death, see chapter 19, Grieving and Accepting the Loss.

10 Conventional Treatments

According to conventional Western veterinary medicine, tumors should be biopsied to determine if they are malignant. This is done to ascertain if cancer is present, what type exists, and whether the animal patient has other health problems. The goal of conventional Western treatment is to eliminate all cancer cells from the body, both at the primary site and at other, more distant sites. According to the Tufts University School of Veterinary Medicine, some cancers can actually be cured[1]—but the word *cure* is defined as the cancer not recurring within a three- to five-year period. This seems quite different from the feelings of the alternative veterinarians I interviewed, most of whom believe that there is no cure for the disease—but that they can treat and help animals with cancer to live longer and more comfortably.

As Samantha Mooney, who worked for several years with cats who had cancer, writes in *A Snowflake in My Hand,* "Cancer is not another word for death. Neither is it a single illness for which there is one cure. Instead it takes many forms, and each form responds differently to treatment."[2]

As I repeat throughout this book, always find a veterinarian or other animal care provider you can trust, one who treats your animal as an individual and is open-minded. As Dr. Myrna Milani reiterated in October 2004, "The most important aspect of this is finding a veterinarian with whom you can communicate well and even under the worst circumstances, if necessary. Given how hectic the average pet owner's life is and the role pets play in that life, it's also important that the veterinarian be sensitive to any owner needs or limits as well as those of the animal."[3]

SURGERY

Surgery is the oldest form of cancer therapy and still the most frequently used, sometimes in conjunction with alternative therapies. Initially it involves a surgical biopsy to make an accurate diagnosis. The complete surgical removal of the tumor is appropriate for most primary tumors. In my experience surgery can often buy an animal months or years of a fairly comfortable life.

According to notes from the North American Veterinary Conference, held in Orlando, Florida, in January 2004: "Surgery is and will remain for the near future the most widely applied modality for cancer control. Surgery can be used for prevention (e.g., ovariohysterectomy before 2.5 years of age), pathology diagnosis including tumor staging, and treatment (cure or palliation)."[4]

Still, Robert C. Rosenthal, D.V.M., explains, "Surgical excision remains the most widely recommended therapy for most tumors, but chemotherapy and other modalities are finding wide application in both the primary and adjunctive settings." Rosenthal believes that as our understanding of using the various techniques together grows, "owners should be offered at least introductory comments on the potential to use more than one means of treating the disease. Such information should lead to improved care for our patients."[5]

Walter Last, the author of *The Self Help Cancer Cure* and *Problem Foods,* notes, however, that surgery leaves cancerous cells behind in 25 to 60 percent of human cancer patients. Malignant growths may recur and, in disrupting the tumor, both the surgery and the preceding biopsy may contribute to cancer's spread in the body.[6]

Donna Raditic, D.V.M., explained to me that a decision to use surgery as a part of treatment is based on several factors: the type of tumor and its location; the known behavior of the cancer; the overall state of health of the patient; the animal guardian's and the patient's wishes (as the guardian can best intuit them); and the economics of the situation. Not all cancers require surgery. Some cancers—for example, lymphosarcoma, the cancer of the lymph system in dogs—do not include surgery as part of their treatment. Surgery may be used both diagnostically and as a "reasonable form of treatment."

But she and many veterinarians feel that surgery is frequently too invasive. "For example, opening a cat's abdomen to obtain a sample of a liver mass is much more invasive than using other techniques such as ultrasound guided needle biopsies." Dr. Raditic rarely performs surgeries for diagnostic purposes only; she tries to find answers with less invasive techniques. And like other holistic veterinarians, she has learned to treat without an exact diagnosis. But she always lets her clients know she is doing this and gives them all their options. In the future, with the help of such tools as CAT scans and nuclear magnetic resonance in veterinary medicine, veterinarians will have a wider range of less invasive tools for making diagnoses.[7]

Anesthesia

Administering anesthesia is potentially life threatening by itself. However, the newest anesthetic drugs are much safer than their predecessors.[8] Veterinarians try to pay close attention to the animal's overall condition and age (older animals need less anesthesia), and to keep the time under anesthesia to a minimum. Animals are treated on an individual basis, as they ought to be for all conditions. Anesthesia does three things: it promotes a loss of consciousness—which includes no memory of what happened; it blocks any painful sensations; and it allows the muscles to relax and suppresses reflexive movement in the patient. Luckily, most animals—cats in particular—awaken headache-free from general anesthetic protocols.[9]

New Types of Surgery

One type of surgical treatment that is becoming more popular and available is laser surgery. The first veterinary use of a laser was in 1971, and since that date laser surgery machines have become more mobile, smaller, and less expensive—dropping from between $60,000 and $150,000 to approximately $25,000.[10] They can now be found in many universities and private veterinary clinics. If your veterinarian does not have one, perhaps he or she knows of one in your geographic area. These beams of light are amazing and quite versatile.

Laser (Light Amplification by Stimulated Emission of Radiation) is being used in more and more human surgeries, outpatient and inpatient. Almost all parts of the body can be treated with lasers effectively and with less pain and sedation than traditional cutting techniques involve.

Lasers are gentler than scalpels in several ways. The laser beam seals blood vessels, so there is much less bleeding. It may be less painful for cats (and other animals), "because the beam seems to cap nerve endings as it cuts, so the cats tolerate the procedure," says Barbara Gores, a board-certified surgeon at Angell Memorial Animal Hospital in Boston. Lasers allow a veterinarian to cut more precisely than with a scalpel. The diseased tissue can be more easily targeted and vaporized; a much smaller area around the tumor can be cut. For example, when a veterinarian removes a benign skin tumor on a cat, he or she can excise only the diseased tissue, without removing any of the surrounding tissue.

Finally, lasers allow a doctor to get into difficult-to-access body parts such as ear canals. Using cats as an example, Dr. Gores explains that with a laser a doctor can preserve the ear canal and the cat's hearing, whereas with a scalpel veterinarians generally have to remove the whole ear canal.[11]

One place where laser surgery is being used successfully is at Timpanogos Animal Hospital in Pleasant Grove, Utah. Three veterinary surgeons there routinely perform a number of procedures with a carbon dioxide laser, including any that involve small masses or tumors. "Pet patients who undergo a declawing, mouth ulcer removal or tumor excision by laser experience noticeably less pain, bleed less and recover more quickly," writes Sharon Haddock.

Explains Darrell Berry, D.V.M., of that facility, "It's a kind of hands-off surgery with less inflammation, less swelling because we've intruded less." He adds that it is "the most humane kind of surgery. I think the laser is going to be used more and more."[12]

DRUG-LASER THERAPY

Another promising pet cancer treatment is drug-laser therapy, a two-part treatment also called photodynamic therapy. The first step is a drug injection, followed by a laser light that activates the chemical. Elsa Beck, D.V.M., a veterinarian in Detroit, explains that photodynamic therapy has been from 40 to 95 percent successful in curing her several hundred patients' cancers, depending on the tumor's location. As a one-time treatment, it has fewer side effects than radiation. Dr. Beck also expresses hope for adapting this type of treatment for use with human cancers: "It's just one of those cases where medicine for man's (and woman's) best friends may also help save human lives."[13]

RADIATION TREATMENTS

Radiation is second in popularity to surgery for use with primary tumors. It is available at veterinary schools and many veterinary hospitals that specialize in cancer treatment. It may be used alone, before or after surgery, or in conjunction with chemotherapy. (However, a veterinary text adds this caution: "A major concern in combining radiation and chemotherapeutic agents is enhanced toxicity to normal tissues. Therefore, drug doses may have to be reduced."[14]) When the risk of complications or physical constraints exist, radiation therapy is often required along with surgery. In the head and limbs radiation therapy might be an alternative to radical surgery. Radiation can also provide relief from symptoms such as pain or bleeding where surgery is not an option. According to Walter Last, radiation rarely cures cancer in humans—and it may cause a large amount of damage and dysfunction in organs and tissues.[15]

Various radiation treatment schedules are offered, such as once a week for three or four treatments; or treatments given three times a week (two days apart each) ten to twelve times over about three weeks. The variations in protocol are meant to minimize hospitalization, to reduce tumor cell repopulation during the treatment, and to limit the amount of anesthesia necessary, because many of the animals in question are elderly and in poor general health. However, some studies have shown that protocols using more treatments with smaller doses of radiation in each produce fewer adverse reactions and result in a better therapeutic gain. When combined with surgery, radiation therapy is given either preoperatively or postoperatively.[16]

According to Michael Walker, D.V.M., veterinarians always think about whether a treatment is a cure or palliation. "Curative radiation therapy, while less common, is possible for certain types [of cancer], but cure is an unrealistic expectation for many tumors." However, he points out that many "incurable" cancers can be treated so that the patient can live longer with a higher quality of life. Palliative radiation therapy might be used in these cases: tumors too large to be "cured," primary or secondary tumors that are painful or obstructing various normal functions, tumors in animals that have coexisting disease, and tumors in dogs or cats whose guardians cannot afford "definitive therapy."[17]

Finally, Dr. Walker says, "Failure to inform clients of what radiation therapy may provide to palliate, if not cure, cancer in an animal may constitute a professional disservice. It is our responsibility to provide adequate information for clients to make informed decisions regarding the health care of their animals."[18]

Side effects of radiation may include fatigue, especially during the last half of therapy, and very occasionally nausea and vomiting. Hair loss in the radiated field will most probably occur, and there may be a change in hair color as it regrows.[19]

New Types of Radiation Therapy

A recent development is a radiation treatment known as brachytherapy, which uses radioactive beads; these are implanted into dogs and cats with certain tumors unlikely to spread throughout their bodies. This treatment has been long used with humans for cervical, breast, endometrial, and, recently, prostate cancer. At Kansas State University (KSU) doctors are using this radiation treatment when surgery cannot be performed or they cannot remove all of the cancerous tumors. Explains Dr. Ruthanne Chun, associate professor of clinical sciences at KSU's veterinary college, "There are maybe two or three other veterinary colleges that do it, so we are really riding the edge of that wave in being able to offer this service."[20]

Once a surgeon has removed as much of the tumor as is possible, he or she sutures a hollow, sterile plastic cube (called an after-loading tube) directly into the tumor-containing organ. The veterinarian closes the wound and inserts the radioactive beads into the after-loading tube. All this is then clamped. The beads emit radiation specifically into the remaining tumor.

Dr. Chun explains that after applying a specific dose, they sedate the animals, remove the tubes and beads, and the therapy is completed. Because the beads provide continuous low-level radiation, the animals are kept in isolation during the procedure and recovery. Anesthesia is needed fewer times than in more conventional forms of radiation, and treatment times are shorter. (Conventional radiation with an external beam unit may require daily anesthesia anywhere from ten to twenty times, which is often quite expensive and hard on the animal.) However, not all tumors can be treated with such an implant at present, and more time is needed to see if animals survive as long as or longer than those treated with other forms of radiation.[21]

Tomotherapy has been in process since July 1995 and is being used in a few practices. This radiation therapy, which means "slice therapy," selectively destroys cancerous tumors while avoiding surrounding healthy tissue. The University of Wisconsin-Madison explains how it works on its Web site: "Tomotherapy rotates the beam source around the patient, thus allowing the beam to enter the patient from many different angles in succession. . . . The tumor is more precisely targeted and the healthy tissue surrounding the tumor is subjected to much lower dosages of radiation."[22] ACT (Animal Cancer Treatment—see page 137), which has recently moved part of its staff to Colorado State University, is using this treatment for canine nasal tumor studies. Although dogs are being treated at the original ACT location, the University of Wisconsin-Madison, they can receive regular follow-ups done at a private practice or other veterinary school elsewhere in the country.[23]

CHEMOTHERAPY

Chemotherapy is now used frequently in many veterinary practices. It works well for patients with systemic cancers such as leukemia and lymphosarcoma. It may be used in combination with surgery and radiation to treat localized high-grade tumors likely to metastasize, or spread. The same chemotherapy drugs used for humans are used for animals, but generally in lower dosages, in fewer combinations, and less frequently. Some are given by mouth; others are injected.[24]

The use of chemotherapy, however, does not come without concerns. One such problem with most chemotherapy, at least in humans, is drug resistance. The majority of cancer cells are genetically unstable and are likely to produce drug-resistant cells.

Human cancer author Walter Last states that in addition, chemotherapy uses toxic drugs that destroy cancer cells—but also attack normal cells. These include bone marrow cells, the foundation of the immune system. "Chemotherapy can drastically undermine the immune system's ability to fight off otherwise harmless bacteria," he writes.[25] Also, chemotherapy-resistant tumorous cells sometimes occur that cause this treatment to fail, and animals, like humans, sometimes experience side effects.[26]

The side effects of chemotherapy may include gastrointestinal toxicity, bone marrow suppression, and immunosuppression (the prevention or diminution of the immune response via irradiation of serums or antibodies), but they are generally less severe in animals than in humans.[27] According to Dr. Dave Reinhard, Assistant Medical Director for Veterinary Pet Insurance, toxicity to the kidneys, heart, or liver can become a concern with the use of chemotherapy in animals.[28] Still, most side effects are temporary and will disappear shortly after the treatment ends. Each course of treatment is designed to fit the patient's medical history—her general health condition and the progression of the disease.[29]

Overall, opinions on the benefits of chemotherapy differ. Earl Mindell, author of many books on human and animal nutrition, offers this reflection: "Chemotherapy and radiation may kill a cancer in the short term, but in the long term the dog's body is severely weakened and her chances of survival are diminished."[30]

According to several owners with dogs who have undergone chemo, the average recovery rate has been only approximately 8 to 10 percent; dogs generally gain only a year of life following this treatment. Still, a year is quite a long time in canine terms, if it can represent quality time.[31]

Veterinarian Donna Raditic once treated a cat with chemotherapy—rare in her practice. This cat apparently did not want the treatment, and the doctors had to anesthetize it before each dose of chemotherapy. "Cats especially have very strong opinions; sometimes they don't want something." Dr. Raditic feels the cat died from the chemotherapy treatments. "I made that cat miserable in its last days. I feel terrible about that."[32] She stresses the importance of learning from such mistakes.

On the other hand, Denise Kessler, D.V.M., is a proponent of the use of chemotherapy in many cases. Her strongest piece of advice for a cat guardian is, "Don't be afraid of chemotherapy. We're encouraging people toward chemotherapy. It's not as bad for animals as for humans. They won't lose their hair. I tell my clients, 'Let's medically treat them until they're well.'"[33]

One issue I did not discuss in my first edition is the use of prednisone, an anti-inflammatory drug, as part of chemotherapy treatment, especially for canine lymphoma. This somewhat controversial drug is often overprescribed to humans, in my humble opinion, for all sorts of things, and has side effects including bloating, excessive thirst, and excessive urination. A friend's young dog who was on prednisone for months was lethargic and had no quality of life. One special concern arises if it is used too long. "When doses become immune-suppressive (higher doses) or use becomes 'chronic' (longer than four months at an every other day schedule), the side effects and concerns associated become different. In these cases, monitoring tests may be recommended or, if possible, another therapy may be selected," write veterinarians at the MarVista Animal Medical Center and Pharmacy.[34] Dr. Myrna Milani has this to say about its use with animals, in general: "Yes, steroids are dangerous but in the overall scheme of things probably no more or less dangerous than any of the chemo agents. . . . With the use of any drug, you always weigh any benefits against possible side effects. . . . The side effects of prednisone are well-known whereas that of many other medications are not. Consequently, it's easier to monitor the patient for them."[35]

New Types of Chemotherapy

One new type of drug treatment involves angiogenesis inhibitors. Angiogenesis is the formation of new blood vessels. The process is controlled by various chemicals produced in the body; these chemicals stimulate the cells to repair weak blood vessels and to form new ones. This process can play an important role in the growth of cancer, because cancer cannot grow or spread without new blood vessels. Scientists are now trying to find ways to stop angiogenesis through both natural and synthetic angiogenesis inhibitors—or anti-angiogenesis agents—in the belief that these chemicals can prevent cancer's growth. In animal experiments angiogenesis inhibitors have already successfully caused the cancer to shrink and die. Side effects and drug resistance may be less pronounced than with standard chemotherapy, because anti-angiogenic drugs target normal, genetically stable cells.[36]

However, this is a very new treatment, and whether it will be equally effective against cancer in people—or in domestic animals—is not yet known. Clinical trials are under way with breast cancers, prostate cancers, lung cancers, ovary and cervix cancers, some leukemias, and more. If the inhibitors prove both safe and effective, they will be approved by the FDA and made available first for humans, as is always the case.[37]

As of July 2004, Dr. Adnan Elfarra, a researcher in the School of Veterinary Medicine, University of Wisconsin-Madison was investigating "prodrugs which can take on the characteristics of an existing cancer drug and selectively deliver it to cancer cells, while sparing normal cells." Existing chemotherapy drugs attack normal as well as cancerous cells. Dr. Elfarra's work is being done on mice; he hopes that results will translate to both human and animal populations.[38]

EXPERIMENTAL TREATMENTS

In addition to the three major treatment approaches (surgery, radiation, and chemotherapy), several experimental treatments are currently being evaluated by veterinarians.

+ *Immunotherapy:* This treatment stimulates an animal's immune system to attack the tumor. Used as part of Immunotherapy, one increasingly popular product, made from colostrum, is Transfer Factor.[39] This product, made by 4Life Research, is used for both animals and humans to boost the immune system. Some veterinarians recommend the human product for animals, according to dozens of testimonials on Shirley's Wellness Cafe, a Web site dedicated to promoting natural health for animals and people.[40]

+ *Hyperthermia:* This is "the raising of tissue temperatures to 42 to 50 degrees C for specific periods of time to produce an antitumor effect," a therapy documented since the time of the ancient Greeks for treatment of tumors. It has been used more popularly with humans since the mid-1900s and is often used with chemotherapy or radiation.[41]

+ *Photodynamic Therapy:* This treatment has had good results on tumors including squamous cell carcinomas, transitional cell carcinomas, and soft-tissue sarcomas.[42]

+ *Bone Transplants:* In dogs, bone transplants have been "reasonably successful and have allowed the pet to avoid amputation," according to Dr. Dave Reinhard, assistant medical director of Veterinary Pet Insurance, the largest pet insurance provider in the United States.

+ *Antisense Therapy:* Antisense drugs are currently in various stages of testing for the treatment of infectious, inflammatory, and cardio-vascular diseases, and cancer in humans. They have actually had some success on prostate cancer. They work by using synthetic DNA or RNA to stop a cell's genetic machinery from producing disease-related proteins. Theoretically, a custom antisense drug could be made to stop any of the two hundred varieties of cancer.[43]

+ *Cryosurgery:* This technique, which destroys tissues by deep freezing, is also occasionally used for some surgeries. It has been used for years in the treatment of human cancers of the liver, prostate, pancreas, and kidney. It is less invasive than conventional surgery and seems to produce fewer complications.[44]

+ *Immuno-Augmentative Therapy (IAT):* This therapy, which straddles the line between conventional and holistic treatments, attempts to redress imbalances in the proteins of the immune system so they can regulate the cancer themselves. Martin Goldstein, D.V.M., one of its primary practitioners, explains it thoroughly in his book, *The Nature of Animal Healing.* It involves analyzing a series of samples of the animal's blood to identify deficiencies, and then addressing those deficiencies with a series of injections. Typically, an animal with cancer receives three to four injections each morning, and the same number in the evening, five days a week. This therapy has an advantage over chemo and radiation in that it is painless and has no side effects.[45]

CONTINUING RESEARCH

Just as for human cancer research, a number of facilities and programs exist that are dedicated to researching this disease in animals.

The ACT Program

An important center for cancer research for animals in the United States, ACT (Animal Cancer Treatment), has been housed in the School of Veterinary Medicine at the University of Wisconsin-Madison for more than twenty years. It was here that Tegan the Irish setter was treated; he lived much longer than originally expected (see chapter 17). Although Tegan is no longer on this planet, he is still on the cover of the program's brochure. Part of the program's staff has recently moved to Colorado State University's Veterinary School but studies will continue in Wisconsin.

The ACT program offers many services, including treatment planning, surgery, chemotherapy, and radiation; a team of board certified oncologists, surgeons, and radiologists work together. As of fall 2004, according to Ilene Kurzman, Associate Scientist at ACT, its research involved the following: tomotherapy for canine nasal tumors; a "phase 1 trial for pegyiated tumor necrosis factor for treatments of canine tumors that have failed traditional therapy or for dogs whose owners have declined traditional therapy; and an allogeneic tumor cell vaccine for treatment of canine melanoma."[46]

This last study is not being funded, so ACT enters dogs into what they term a "compassionate use" study; the animal guardian must pay all bills. This is a nationwide program; any veterinarian throughout the country can administer the vaccine. Explains Kurzman, "The bottom line on this study is people find out that we have a vaccine, call me to talk about the protocol, and if they want to try it. I then arrange to ship it to their veterinarian. The owner needs to contact me to set this up."[47]

Finally, a new study began this past January 2005. This centers on a new chemotherapy drug for canine mast cell tumors. "This study is for dogs with disease at stage 2 or higher," explained Kurzman.[48] Clinical trials are open for referrals from all over the United States— and the center has an excellent national reputation. The fees include treatments and follow-up in most cases. For more information, the Veterinary Medical Teaching Hospital referral coordinator can be reached at (608) 262-7676 or (800) DVM-VMTH.[49]

AN OPPOSING VIEW OF THE TOP THREE

Surgery, chemotherapy, and radiation are widely used and should be considered in many cases. However, homeopathic veterinarian Richard Pitcairn says this about conventional treatments: "Though chemotherapy, radiation and surgery can have dramatic and rapid results, the quality of life for the animals afterwards does not impress me. Life is more than just physical duration. To me it is not enough for the patient to be alive—there must also be some pleasure in that life. From the beginning of my career in veterinary medicine, I have been averse to the harsh treatments used for cancer. It just doesn't feel right to me." He also feels that conventional treatments are not especially effective for prolonging life. "Considering the discomfort entailed in conventional treatment, I don't think it is worth it."[50]

A famous doctor for humans, Andrew Weil, shares these feelings about chemotherapy and radiation: "I have always believed that chemotherapy and radiation as we know it will eventually become obsolete cancer treatments." Rather, he believes experimental therapies including immunotherapy, the Hoxsey Treatment (see chapter 12, Herbs and Bach Flower Remedies), and others ought to be further considered in use for human cancers.[51]

If you opt for giving your pet conventional treatments, Dr. Pitcairn recommends these measures to help support the body during these procedures: Feed only fresh, unprocessed foods; only organic meat if possible. Give high levels of vitamin C. Give oat tincture. Use only spring-, distilled, or other pure water. Feed cooked oatmeal and give the homeopathic remedy Nux Vomica 6C if the animal becomes ill from the drugs. And avoid all vaccinations.[52] (See chapter 8, Vaccinations, for more on Dr. Pitcairn's views on this.)

Another viewpoint comes from R. M. Clemmons, D.V.M.: "To me, the answer to cancer lies in the immune system. This is the major reason why I have trouble with Western chemotherapy. Spontaneous remission from cancer only occurs when the patient's immune system acts to clear the cancer. Therefore, stimulation of the patient's immune system to selectively attack the cancer seems to be the key to achieving a successful outcome. New methods in immunotherapy and immunotargeted chemotherapy are likely to be the Western methods which lead to the greatest advances in cancer treatment over the next few decades."[53] He also nods to traditional Eastern medicine as an approach to combine with Western techniques to help heal patients. "An integrative approach combining the best of both Western and Eastern medicine seems to be the only sensible course of action, providing the best overall care for the patient."[54]

11 An Introduction to Alternative Therapies

As is true in human medicine, alternative therapies are becoming more popular in veterinary health care. This is true even in the case of large animals; acupuncture is being used increasingly in horse treatments. An increasing number of practitioners are using alternative modalities along with the more conventional treatments to offer a full spectrum of services to their animal patients—and to fill their human clients' desires and requests. Use of the term *alternative* is somewhat controversial; many veterinarians prefer the terms *holistic, complementary,* or *integrative.*

According to Myrna M. Milani, D.V.M., in her book *The Art of Veterinary Practice,* studies have indicated that as of 1993 as much as 37 percent of the American public sought out alternative treatments. As a rule, these people tend to be more highly educated and more affluent than average.[1] Dr. Milani notes that many individuals seek out alternatives for their animal companions because they have lost faith in the treatment, *not* because they have lost faith in their longtime doctor.

However, alternative therapies have still not caught on in the United States as readily as they have in many other countries. States Milani, "It's very gratifying to know that the awareness of the connection between health, behavior, and the bond is growing, no matter how slowly." Dr. Milani reports that she has received very few requests from clients for alternative treatments. She believes "The problem is that all the alternatives were developed on a philosophy of helping the mind-body heal itself and that takes time and commitment, both of which may not fit the quick-fix mentality of our society."[2]

Based on my research, those alternative treatments most widely accepted and used today are acupuncture; dietary changes tending toward more natural or homemade; use of more vitamins, minerals, and herbs; and homeopathic treatments. Western Europeans, Australians, and Canadians seem to be more accepting of these treatments and seem to have incorporated these treatments more fully than we in the United States. On a trip to France in the fall of 2004, I was happy to note that most pharmacies carried homeopathic or herbal treatments.

Acceptance in the United States is changing as well. When I speak of alternative treatments to my friends, neighbors, and colleagues, many of them have tried either acupuncture or dietary changes. Many of them are cutting back on the number of vaccines they give to their dogs or cats. And many, too, have offered their animal companions chemotherapy or radiation rather than just let them go downhill after a couple of surgeries. I know that these latter treatments are not alternative, but they are still relatively new—and not well known—to the entire population of animal lovers. People are, in general, willing to do more and spend more money on their animal companions' health these days. They are not willing to accept only the options of surgery or euthanasia.

In *The Nature of Animal Healing: The Path to Your Pet's Health, Happiness, and Longevity*, Martin Goldstein, D.V.M., defines *holistic medicine* this way: "Holistic medicine is nothing if not a therapy of hope: until an animal actually dies, there's hope of recovery from even the direst condition, because when you allow for miracles by persisting with the right natural supplements, sometimes they occur." He states that a basic principle of alternative practices is "that there are no coincidences."[3]

Randy Kidd, president of the American Holistic Veterinary Medical Association (AHVMA), finds that "People are seeing good results with alternative medicine on themselves, and they want the same thing for their pets." Kidd also notes that the interest in holistic pet care has prompted a few veterinary schools to add short courses on such topics as acupuncture and homeopathy.[4]

According to Theresa M. Mall, secretary to the executive director of the AHVMA, their group now has 700+ members in the United States and more than 55 internationally, including many in Canada. "Our membership rate has leveled in the last few years, though this year has been better than the last two," she wrote me.[5]

Edward C. Boldt Jr., D.V.M., executive director of the International Veterinary Acupuncture Society (IVAS), recently told me the group currently has approximately 1250 members, and that number increases each year. Members come from around the world and courses are taught in the United States, Britain, Norway, Belgium, and Australia. The majority of the certified members also offer conventional veterinary medicine.[6]

Dr. Milani says that many veterinarians decide to offer alternative treatments because they see that the old ones do not work in all cases. If veterinarians see their purpose as helping animals regain and maintain their health, rather than just completing the process of conventional treatments, then it "seems that any treatment which accomplishes that purpose is valid." Most veterinarians choose to look to alternative therapies for two reasons, Milani notes: The conventional approaches are not working in a particular type of case; or the client requests an alternative therapy.[7] Perhaps that client has done some reading or has heard positive reports about some therapy from friends or family. Milani believes that most veterinarians do not use alternatives "to flout the system," but instead find themselves in situations where they have done everything else and the animal is not improving.

She notes that, as with all treatments, "the probability of any alternative curing an animal is fifty-fifty: it either works or it doesn't." But she points out wisely that treatments may work in less obvious ways: for example, sometimes a veterinarian's willingness to try new techniques may help the client keep the animal alive a bit longer, even if the disease is not truly cured.[8]

One of the problems that may arise is that you, the caregiver, may want your veterinarian to try some alternative treatments, but he or she may not want to do so. This can happen for a number of reasons. The vet may not believe in them or may not have the expertise to offer them. This can pose an ethical and moral problem for some doctors. However, as Dr. Milani notes (and I heartily agree), veterinarians ought to at least listen to your requests and try not to dismiss the less traditional treatments out of hand. Milani is clear that practitioners should not do anything that violates their belief system, but she does believe it makes sense for them to at least recognize their clients' beliefs as different *rather than wrong*. Rather than alienate their clients, they should be able to explain why they don't believe in or trust the alternative treatments. In many cases they could also refer owners to a veterinarian who does believe in these treatments and has the expertise to perform them.[9]

According to veterinarian Richard C. Swanson, president of the American Veterinary Medical Association (the animal health care profession's version of the AMA), his organization issued guidelines in 1996 on the use of alternative and complementary treatments in veterinary medicine. "There is evidence that acupuncture is probably effective for certain conditions," he notes, such as chronic pain. He also believes that chiropractic seems to help small animals.[10]

In a nutshell these guidelines state:

+ Veterinary acupuncture and acutherapy received the highest vote of confidence. These should be regarded as surgical and/or medical procedures.
+ Veterinarians should undertake educational programs to practice veterinary acupuncture.
+ In the case of chiropractic, research is limited; further research is recommended. Veterinary chiropractic should be performed by licensed veterinarians, or if a state's practice acts permit, licensed chiropractors educated in veterinary chiropractic may be allowed to do so under the supervision of or referral by a licensed veterinarian also involved in the case.
+ Regarding homeopathy, "clinical and anecdotal evidence exists to indicate that veterinary homeopathy may be beneficial." However, further research and education are recommended. Since "some of these substances may be toxic," only licensed veterinarians educated in these methods should perform such treatments.[11]

One clear indication that alternative medicine is becoming more popular to consumers is the success of AltVetMed, a huge Web site run by two veterinarians, Jan A. Bergeron, V.M.D., and Susan G. Wynn,

D.V.M. This site (www.altvetmed.org) contains dozens of links and lots of current information on alternative and complementary therapies. Begun in January 1996, it has been listed in a number of national publications. In March 1997 an article on the CNN Web site included a link to AltVetMed.[12] In addition, the number of visitors to the site is steadily climbing. Dr. Bergeron reports that "the pattern is one of increased visitors reflecting increased interest in alternative medicine for animals."[13]

However, Dr. Wynn, who has also coauthored (with Allen M. Schoen, D.V.M.) *Complementary and Alternative Veterinary Medicine Principles and Practice,* says, "Can't natural treatments alone cure cancer? . . . In a word, no. What natural treatments can do is improve the animal's general state of health and give it a better chance to fight the disease." In fact, she is not against chemotherapy for some cancers, especially lymphoma, which responds well to this treatment. She notes that other cancers, such as primary lung carcinomas or melanomas, generally have a variable or poor response to drugs. She adds, "No controlled trials comparing the two approaches (conventional or surgery, and the like versus holistic) have ever been done."[14]

In a more recent statement, Dr. Wynn writes, "It is extremely important that the holistic veterinarian be presented with the entire history, and given more patience than is expected in an emergency room, or a strictly western medicine hospital environment." She stresses the importance of clients bearing with their integrative holistic veterinarians, as they review the history, lab work, and other diagnostic work and decide on the "most appropriate complementary therapies" because this may require some longer period of time.[15]

12 Herbs and Bach Flower Remedies

Herbalism and Bach flower therapy are two forms of alternative treatment gaining in popularity as people look more and more to the natural world for the means to support their ill animals. In searching for ways to help a pet who has been diagnosed with cancer, many are turning to the potential power of plants to ease discomfort, boost immunity, and soothe emotional stress.

HERBS

The use of herbs is one of the oldest forms of medicine in the world. Herbs have been given to animals for centuries in societies that value creatures highly. According to Susan G. Wynn, D.V.M., "Prehistoric people may have found therapeutic principles by trial and error, or perhaps by watching animals 'treat' themselves by eating special plants when ill."[1]

In an article in the popular magazine *Time,* writer Christine Gorman says that alternative treatments, including herbs and acupuncture, are increasingly popular with animal guardians, at least in the United States. According to Gorman's findings, alternative medicine is more supported for animal companions than it is for humans among those in the medical community. A few of the more popular herbs being used are echinacea, clove, and Irish moss to boost the potency of the immune system. Herbs are also used in diluted preparations in home-opathy to combat cancer and other diseases.[2]

According to the editors of *A Passion for Dogs: The Dogs Home Battersea,* herbs are used to treat a variety of conditions in dogs. The editors feel that all herbal remedies are safe if used correctly, but implore readers to be sure the dose used is many times smaller than that which could cause any harm. They stress that variations need to be made for breed, age, and the strength of the patient—and also for the condition and the stage of the illness.[3]

As is true with a human patient, when a holistic doctor evaluates an animal's condition, all the problems and individual idiosyncrasies of the patient will be considered, not just the presenting disease (in this case, cancer). Practitioners may use combinations of herbs to treat symptoms. Dr. Wynn says that combinations may have two advantages: the therapeutic principles are concentrated by the "synergy," the addi-tive effects of the group of herbs; and any toxic effect in one herb may be diluted by the other herbs. However, she points out that doses and protocols are not formalized in veterinary herbal medicine. It is not always safe to base prescriptions proportionally by comparing them to human body weights. For example, while white willow is commonly used to relieve human arthritic pain, if you attempted to treat an arthritic cat with a smaller dose of it, she could die. Cats cannot metab-olize the salicylic acid contained in the plant.

Mild herbs, such as raspberry for pregnancy, milk thistle for hepa-titis, and echinacea for immune stimulation, have been used on animals for years with no adverse side effects.[4]

According to Richard H. Pitcairn, D.V.M., in his seminal *Dr. Pitcairn's Complete Guide to Natural Health for Dogs and Cats,* herbal remedies have long been used for a variety of illnesses in animals. These include treating dogs for worms, fleas, skin problems, kidney and blad-der ailments, wounds and fractures, warts, and more. In his practice and his books, Dr. Pitcairn prefers to emphasize homeopathic medica-tions, which "generally taste good and are given less frequently," to straight fresh herbs. He also uses some Bach flower remedies. "I find [herbs] most useful for external treatments on animals or for minor upsets that do not require prolonged treatment," he writes in the latest edition of his book.[5]

In an article, "Herbs for Animals," from the Veterinary Botanical Medicine Association, its writers state, "It is unwise to assume that herbs alone are used to treat ill-health in our pets. Most holistic veterinarians recommend nutritional support, in addition to conventional therapy if the problem is acute, severe or life threatening." They recommend garlic and turmeric for cancer treatment and shitake mushrooms as an immune stimulant. However, they advise consulting a veterinary herbalist before using herbs for your sick animal.[6]

Herbalist Robert McDowell, N.D., of Australia, who works with dogs, cats, and horses, feels no conflict in combining conventional and herbal treatments. "Although, after I have demonstrated a remission or a reversal [with the use of herbs and dietary changes]," he says "I strongly recommend ceasing ongoing or follow-up chemo or radiotherapy, as these treatments are so destructive to the immune system itself."[7]

ARTEMISININ

Since the first edition of this book appeared, much research has been done on artemisinin, an ancient Chinese medicinal herb, also called wormwood. This medicinal herb was rediscovered in an archeological dig in the 1970s. In a tomb of a prince of the Han Dynasty, was discovered a treatise, "Medical Treatments for 52 Diseases," including advice about using the artemisia herb as a treatment for malaria. In 1972, wormwood's active compound was discovered to be artemisinin.

This herb has been successful in treating malaria for many years, but two researchers, Henry Lai and Nardndra Singh of the University of Washington, have since reported that "artemisinin kills breast cancer cells selectively with only minimal impact on normal breast cells," states veterinarian Narda G. Robinson, D.O., D.V.M., of Colorado State University Veterinary Teaching Hospital, in her article, "Treatment Covers Malaria and Cancer." In one nonhuman study with artemisinin, "within five days of treatment the dog [who could not walk at all] was able to walk normally, and X-rays confirmed the disappearance of the tumor." Other dogs with lymphosarcoma treated with artemisinin saw an immediate reduction in their tumor's size."

Although minimal adverse effects have been found for the herb's antimalarial activity, these do not necessarily mean the same for anti-cancer treatment in dogs and cats. "How safe, then, is this anti-cancer 'smart bomb' for dogs?" asks Robinson. She is somewhat cautionary, believing that veterinary clients need accurate toxicity information and adding that vets in some U.S. states are not covered under professional liability insurance for prescribing herbs such as this.[8] However, according to all reports I have uncovered, this herb deserves further examination and consideration.

ESSIAC

An herbal remedy sometimes found to be effective in the treatment of cancer is Essiac. This is an herbal decoction (or tea) named for Renée Caisse, a nurse from Ontario, Canada. (The word *Essiac* is her name spelled backward.) In 1922 she received a formula that had originated with an Ojibway medicine from a patient who had successfully treated her own breast cancer. Caisse's aunt developed "terminal" cancer, and the physician agreed to let her try the formula. The aunt lived for twenty years, while Caisse eventually opened a clinic and did not charge patients for treatment.

Many doctors, however, did not like the idea of a nurse treating patients. A legal battle ensued. In 1937 the Royal Cancer Commission conducted hearings about Essiac; Parliament was pushed by the population (and by some doctors) to legalize its use. The vote was taken in 1938, but Essiac failed to achieve approval by three votes. After this Caisse closed her Canadian clinic.

In the 1960s Nurse Caisse worked with Dr. Charles Brusch (JFK's physician) at the Brusch Clinic in Massachusetts. Brusch is known to have said, "Essiac is a cure for cancer, period. All studies in the United States and Canada support this conclusion."

Fourteen months before her death Caisse released the ingredients of Essiac to a Canadian company, Resperin. The properties now belong to Essiac Products, and the product is marketed by Essiac International of Canada.[9]

The remedy has been used by herbalists to treat many human cancers—brain, bone, eye, ovarian, and more. Essiac helps detoxify the body of excess mucus, heavy metals, and toxic waste. It also improves liver function, acts as an antioxidant, and strengthens both the pancreas and the spleen. The immune system is greatly strengthened, which helps in healing.[10] The four ingredients, finally available to the public, are also classified as food items: burdock root, sheep sorrel, slippery elm, and turkey rhubarb or rhubarb root. It is the sheep sorrel that contains the cancer-destroying properties. Walter Last, author of *The Self Help Cancer Cure*, warns, however, that some distributors have substituted yellow dock or curly dock for this essential ingredient.[11] Neal K. Weiner, D.V.M., discusses this formula's use for diabetes: "I'll often use Essiac tea. . . . It's a powerful detoxifier and immune-system strengthener. I show my clients how to brew the tea, and they mix it in with the dog's food."[12]

Clare E. Middle, B.V.M.S., of Australia has been using Essiac (now called Can-T in that country) with animals for some time. Over the past two years she has treated more than twenty animals with the herbal mixture, among them "budgies with lumps, a guinea pig with mammary cancer, and many dogs and cats." She has told me that the Australian government is currently reviewing both human and veterinary use of Essiac, and three eminent oncology centers in Europe—the Leornadis Clinic in Germany, the Dobling Sanatorium in Vienna, Austria, and the University of Cologne in Germany—are doing research with human patients. Dr. Middle frequently uses Essiac as an alternative to chemotherapy and has had some success. In the summer of 1998 the Australian government made Can-T available on the open market, so "we don't have to sneak it in as an import any more!"[13]

The Essiac she uses comes in the form of a dry powder, which is boiled up twice by the client and stored in a two-liter container in the refrigerator. Cats receive direct oral dosages of 5 milliliters, and up to 60 milliliters can be used for a large dog. For especially serious cases Dr. Middle gives the recommended maximum dose four times daily for three weeks, rather than twice a day (the original protocol). Cost can be a factor here: Treating a large dog four times a day for three weeks could cost $200. In her practice animals generally take Essiac by syringe or lap it up in milk, soup, or vegetable broth. She does not advise giving it within an hour of eating more solid food.

In Dr. Middle's twenty cases, including dogs, cats, and a canary, all but two had a thorough workup that resulted in the diagnosis of a malignancy. According to both guardian and doctor, more than half of the animals showed demonstrable improvement after using Essiac. Within days of the Essiac treatment they felt better; they also "survived better quality and longer lives than would have been expected with no treatment." After one year, seven of the animals were still alive "and bright and active." Many of the cases also received other natural therapies, including flower essences and homeopathic aids. Diet and nutritional support were tackled when necessary and appropriate. Although the animals did not live many years longer, they did, in more than half the cases, live happier remaining lives. "A lot of healing can be achieved in these times even if cure is not," writes Dr. Middle. Still, she admits of Joe, a six-year-old Dalmatian-cross male dog with lymphosarcoma, that "this swift and peaceful death can sometimes be a feature of natural therapies treatment."[14]

GARLIC

Garlic has been given medicinally to both humans and animals for at least four thousand years. For example, the Egyptians swore on a clove of garlic when taking an oath; Egyptian pharaohs were entombed with carvings of garlic; Egyptian slaves ate garlic while building the pyramids.[15] In the past twenty years two thousand studies have been performed on garlic's impact on our most serious, widespread illnesses. One report concluded that the herb may have direct benefits against the "seven major diseases of our time": hypertension, hyperlipemia (high cholesterol), heavy metal intoxication, infectious disease, free-radical damage, cancer, and immune deficiency disease.

The National Cancer Institute has developed a Designer Foods Program, a five-year study attempting to identify foods that may prevent cancer and prevent cells from becoming cancerous. According to the article "Cancer-Fighting Botanicals" by Braddock Ray, the National Cancer Institute research has found garlic to be effective in inhibiting the growth of cancer cells. North Americans observed that in China the population in a garlic-consuming area had the country's lowest death rate from stomach cancer; people in a nearby country who ate little garlic had thirteen times the mortality rate from this disease. Also, in Italy studies have shown an inverse relationship between cooked garlic and stomach cancer risk.[16] According to Walter Last's research, garlic protects against metastases and inhibits the growth of existing tumors. It also strengthens the immune system and allows the liver to detoxify more effectively.[17]

Here is one example of how this plays out in animals: cats' immune systems can easily become compromised; among the causes are poor diet, stress, disease, breeding and showing, and even aging. Garlic is one herb that can help rebuild the immune system. It has been shown, through a variety of experiments, to be effective against viral infections, parasites, and fungal infections. It is sometimes used to treat fleas, but only the real, fresh item; garlic salt and garlic flavoring do not work at all.[18] One drawback is that it may cause anemia if given for long periods of time.

Rex and Christine Munday, husband and wife researchers from New Zealand, looked at a key ingredient in garlic: diallyl disulfide, which causes the gut to produce enzymes that can clear it of cancer-causing particles. In a study performed on rats, they found that benefits kicked in at between 0.075 and 0.3 milligram of disulfide per kilogram of body weight, or half a clove of garlic for an average-sized human. Diallyl disulfide was first proven to slow the growth of bowel cancer in 1995. A researcher at Pennsylvania State University, Dr. Sujatha Sundaram, found that the substance caused human bowel cancer tumor cells to shrink and die when they were transplanted into mice. He also found another compound in garlic that slowed the progress of breast cancer in rats.[19]

In her 1999 book, *Keep Your Dog Healthy the Natural Way*, medical writer Pat Lazarus lists garlic as one of several nutritional supports for canine cancer patients. Based on veterinarians' reports, she recommends garlic tablets (Garlkicin or Kyolic); give one tablet daily to a small dog, two to three tablets twice daily to a larger dog.[20]

HOXSEY TREATMENT

One of the most fascinating stories of herbs and the treatment of animal and human cancer started with a horse finding its own cure! This is the story of the Hoxsey Treatment, considered one of the "longest-lived unconventional therapies of this century."[21] It is still being used at the Bio-Medical Center of Tijuana, Mexico, but it was first introduced in the early part of the century.

Harry Hoxsey (1909–74) was an Illinois coal miner who was bequeathed an herbal remedy developed in the mid-nineteenth century by his horse breeder great-grandfather, John Hoxsey. According to Harry's report, one of John Hoxsey's favorite stallions, who had a cancerous growth, grazed daily on a variety of wild plants. John reasoned that these wild plants caused the stallion's eventual recovery. He then concocted a liquid (for internal treatments) out of red clover, alfalfa, buckthorn, prickly ash, and a few other plants that he did not know, adding ingredients from old folk remedies for cancer until he made an herbal mixture that seemed also to help other afflicted horses on his Illinois farm. He subsequently developed an external treatment as well, a pasty treatment that included bloodroot, which had long been used by Native American healers to treat cancer.

According to great-grandson Harry's autobiography, John Hoxsey's reputation brought him horses from all over Illinois and from as far away as Kentucky and Indiana. The secret formula was passed along to Harry's father, John, a veterinary surgeon licensed under the Illinois Medical Practice Act. The father began to treat human patients with this mixture as well. Beginning at the age of eight Harry worked as his father's assistant; eventually their human patient load grew to be larger than their animal.[22]

In the 1950s, in the midst of court litigations, Hoxsey publicly revealed his formula. Writes Patricia Ward Spain, who was commissioned by the Office of Technology Assessment of the U.S. Congress to write a report, "He explained that, depending on the type and stage of cancer, and the individual patient's condition, he added a basic solution of cascara and potassium iodide to one or more of the following plant substances: poke root; burdock root; barberry or berberis root; buckthorn bark; Stillingia root; and prickly ash bark."[23]

By the 1950s Hoxsey's clinic in Dallas was the world's largest privately owned cancer center, with branches in seventeen states. Hoxsey not only believed in his unique herbal mixture but he also practiced immunotherapy, some chemotherapy, homeopathy, and chelation therapy. The types of cancer that respond best to the original Hoxsey therapy are reportedly lymphoma, melanoma, and external skin cancers.[24]

But Hoxsey was and still is considered a quack by many, especially those who require strict scientific evidence to support a remedy's claims. According to a report from the Bio-Medical Center itself, "Many of the herbs or the isolated components of these herbs have shown to have anticancer effects in test animals. However, the complete Hoxsey herbal mixture has not been tested for antitumor activity in animals, human cells in culture, or in humans." A congressional study on alternative cancer therapies did not support the tonic's efficacy.[25] Still, some more recent orthodox scientific researchers have identified antitumor properties in all but three of Hoxsey's plants.[26]

The clinic still exists in Mexico, a site that Hoxsey chose in 1963. After his death, his longtime assistant, Mildred Nelson, R.N., ran it until she died in 1999. (Hoxsey had treated Nelson's mother for cancer, and she survived longer than expected.) Now Nelson's sister, Liz Jonas, who has worked at the center since 1996, runs the treatment facility and continues the work for humans with cancer. Patients continue to come from around the world, often after surgery, radiation, and chemotherapy have failed to effectively treat the disease.

Andrew Weil, M.D., author of *8 Weeks to Optimal Health* and *Health and Healing*, is on record as saying of the Hoxsey Treatment: "In my opinion it should be studied."[27]

The remedy that began with a horse's discovery is now primarily confined to human use. Kenny Ausubel, author of the new book *When Healing Becomes a Crime*, says, "While Mildred [Nelson] was alive, she did treat some [animals], and I personally have heard several stories of animals being cured, such as a terminally cancerous dog put on the tonic. . . . [However,] Mildred never promoted this fact because it could deluge the clinic with pets instead of people."[28]

OTHER HERBS

An herb that Russell Swift, D.V.M., recommends for some animal uses is milk thistle, which is especially effective for liver problems. The herb stimulates protein synthesis; helps protect the liver against poison; inhibits the formation of inflammatory substances; helps the liver break down toxins; and is a potent antioxidant. "This means it can counteract free radical damage that can cause degenerative diseases including cancer," Dr. Swift writes. Milk thistle also increases intracellular levels of glutathione, necessary for detoxicating reactions. Swift recommends using the whole herb or a high-quality extract, preferring a standardized product (70 to 80 percent silybin, the best-known active ingredient). He writes that if an animal has been medicated with such substances as antibiotics, cortisone, chemotherapy, antiseizure medications, and others, or has had other liver problems, a course of milk thistle may help. He also indicates that it is important to reduce your animal companion's exposure to liver-toxic substances in her environment, such as poisonous mushrooms, heavy metals, and alcohol.[29]

Another veterinarian, R. M. Clemmons, states that milk thistle may protect the liver from damage by chemotherapy in humans, and may help prevent damage from traditional anticonvulsants.[30]

Dr. Pitcairn believes that goldenseal *(Hydrastis canadensis)* is generally helpful for treating any kind of cancer, especially those varieties that result in weight loss. He always recommends using freshly harvested and dried herbs if possible—the newer, the better. Tinctures are useful because they maintain potency for at least two years, sometimes longer. Gelatin capsules help preserve powdered herbs and help them stay fresh by excluding oxygen, which degrades their effectiveness. In *Dr. Pitcairn's Complete Guide to Natural Health for Dogs and Cats,* the author gives six schedules, both internal and external, that list the frequency and form of herb to be given. However, he cautions that you will need to supplement your animal's diet with extra vitamin B complex when using this herb over long periods of time.[31]

But goldenseal, which is primarily used to fight infection, has become scarce in its native North American habitat due to overharvesting and habitat destruction. It grows most commonly in the Alleghenies in Ohio, Indiana, West Virginia, and Kentucky. Goldenseal is currently one of numerous wild medicinal plants considered at risk by United Plant Savers, a Vermont-based nonprofit group.[32] Purchasing cultivated rather than wild goldenseal is recommended by most herbalists. In addition, writer Becky Gillette says, "Unlike echinacea, there are no scientific studies confirming the medicinal properties attributed to goldenseal."[33]

According to one respected company that sells organically grown herbs for both human and animal use, Avena Botanicals of Rockport, Maine,

"Animals have always relied on plants for food and medicine. . . . Yet . . . most animals are unable to run freely, are bathed in toxic chemicals, and are fed commercial foods containing artificial preservatives and hormones." The results are increases in various diseases, including cancer. Herbalists at Avena believe that "offering animals herbs is a way to help reconnect them with their natural environment." They sell a variety of tinctures for use with animals and also make referrals to homeopathic vets. Products include Calendula Oil, Herbal Supplement for Animals; Daily Tonic for Animals; and more.[34]

Dr. Pitcairn uses herbs as transitional aids when switching an animal from a commercial pet food to a homemade, more natural one. If your dog or cat becomes distressed when changing diets or refuses to eat, a few herbs can help cleanse the body and rebuild tissues. Pitcairn recommends using only one at a time, not a combination. A few he recommends are alfalfa to stimulate digestion and appetite; burdock for cleaning the blood and detoxifying the body; garlic to promote intestinal health; oats as a tonic and as a cleanser (he recommends using them as the major grain in the new diet); and oat straw boiled in water as a healing bath. He also uses the latter for many external problems including skin irritations and aches and pains.[35]

Writers and herbalists Gregory L. Tilford and Mary Wulff-Tilford (who own Animals' Apawthecary and are authors of many books, including *All You Ever Wanted to Know about Herbs for Pets*) recommend a variety of herbs for cats, including some for health purposes and others more for pleasure, such as catnip. Prominent on their list is echinacea, which, of course, has been also gaining popularity among humans in the past decade or so. They write that echinacea "supports healthy immune functions by stimulating and strengthening them at several levels in the body."[36] Most herbalists feel that the herb's complex structure is made up of a therapeutic synergy, but, according to Tilford and Wulff-Tilford, many studies have identified the herb's most influential immune system boosting aids as "an extensive array of components, including caffeic acids, volatile oils, polysaccharides, polyenes, polyines and isobutylamides." These two writers, who have worked with veterinarians for years, prefer to use low-alcohol, glycerine extracts with animals. These extracts do not make the tongue tingle quite so much and include a sweet taste of vegetable glycerine. Their conservative rule for cats is to give ten drops of an herbal tincture, three times a day. However, they caution not to use echinacea on animals with abnormal immune functions. If given to animals with diseases that cause the immune system to work against itself, echinacea may aggravate the disease. Like most herbal experts, they advise consulting your holistic veterinarian before using this herb.[37]

Your kitty herbal cabinet should also include bugleweed, catnip, couchgrass or quackgrass, ginkgo biloba, hawthorn, licorice, marsh mallow, nettle, and skullcap. Mary Wulff-Tilford relates that animals may need more frequent dosages of herbal tinctures than humans because they have higher metabolisms. The two herbalists believe that herbs are best used for five days and then given a rest so the body will not become too accustomed to them.[38]

Dr. Clemmons lists pau d'arco as a helpful herb to use for some canine cancers. This is an extract from the inner bark of South American rain forest trees in the *Tahebuia* genus. The bark contains lapachol, reported to induce strong biological activity in cancer cells yet have no adverse effects on the body. Clemmons points to studies with pure lapachol that also attribute its effectiveness to phytochemicals in the extract. This herbal extract is helpful for humans as well as dogs.[39]

According to literature from Lisa Ayala, a certified herbalist and iridologist, pau d'arco is given out free of charge by the Argentinean government to cancer and leukemia patients.[40] It has shown antitumor effects against mouse Walder 256 carcinoma, Yoshida sarcoma, and Murphy-Sturm lymphosarcoma. However, writes David McCluggage, D.V.M., some clinical trials in people have not shown it to be effective; patients also developed side effects including anemia, nausea, vomiting, and anticoagulant activity. In a study of nineteen patients who received lapachol, only one experienced partial regression of the tumor. Although Dr. McCluggage states that it is considered a strong immune system booster, "there has not been enough clinical evidence to prove its efficacy in cancer therapy.[41]

An additional herbal remedy Dr. Clemmons notes for use with dogs is, ironically, named cat's claw (its name is derived from thorns on the vines). Another rain forest plant, this one from Peru, it was traditionally used by indigenous people for cancer and arthritis. Studies have indicated that it contains immune-enhancing substances, such as antioxidant compounds, which may give it antitumor properties. Some treatments have led to remission of brain and other tumors. Clemmons admits that although published data is unavailable, cat's claw could likely be considered for tumors of the central nervous system.[42]

Martin Goldstein, D.V.M., famous for his treatment of animal cancer patients, believes that your pets can use aloe vera juice either orally (for intestinal function, constipation, or chronic diarrhea), or externally (for burns, rashes, and stings).[43] Aloe vera originated in Africa; about two hundred varieties exist. Most commercial aloe vera is now grown in Caribbean areas, and in Central and South America. The plant has a long history of use for health purposes, especially for treating burns and wounds. It is probably the most famous herbal remedy known to humans.

One study has shown that aloe vera may stop immune system damage caused by sunburn, perhaps making it useful in the treatment of skin cancers. Other researchers have reported that some substances in the herb reduce inflammation and stimulate the growth of white blood cells and other cells connected with immune functions.[44] In one of the more persuasive studies, a researcher "found that fresh aloe vera leaves contained lectin like compounds which enhanced the growth of normal human cells in tissue culture, but not tumor cells." Earlier studies also confimed that while aloe vera does promote regeneration of normal tissue, it does not do this with carcinogenic tissue. Many of the scientific studies have commented that it is probably the synergistic effect of the compounds in the plant that accounts for these healing activities.[45]

Aloe vera has even been licensed by the USDA for treating cancer, by injection, in dogs and cats. According to Ian Tizard, veterinary pathobiologist at Texas A&M University, aloe vera works best to accelerate wound-healing in animal patients. He is conducting research on the plant, which he states demonstrates almost a total lack of toxicity, reduces inflammation from radiation therapy, and is a great wound healer for the elderly.[46]

In her popular book *Four Paws Five Directions: A Guide to Chinese Medicine for Cats and Dogs,* Cheryl Schwartz, D.V.M., praises the use of herbs in the treatment of cancer for three reasons. They can act as the first line of defense in "debilitated, older animals" or be used with chemotherapy or radiation therapy, to help "strengthen the individual and mitigate side effects." Herbs also can effectively treat pain, and are more easily tolerated by animals who are drug sensitive.[47]

MUSHROOMS

One herb Cheryl Schwartz mentions is ganoderma mushrooms, which appear to stop the spread of some tumors.[48] The ganoderma mushroom, or reishi, is a medicinal mushroom from Asia. It meets all the qualifications of being both a tonic and an adaptogen—strengthening and invigorating organs, and helping the body adapt to stress. Chinese scientists have conducted many studies of reishi. It appears to strengthen the immune system by preventing a variety of diseases and conditions, including but not limited to allergies, insomnia, and some cancers. Reishi and other mushrooms such as shiitake and maitake can significantly lower serum cholesterol and thin the blood, much as aspirin does. Reishi has also been studied for its ability to curtail high blood pressure in the human animal. Even when taken in large quantities by humans (350 grams per day for thirty days), it is unlikely to have a toxic effect.[49]

These mushrooms are also considered to "calm the spirit, protect and clear heat from the central nervous system, open the heart . . . lower blood pressure, [they] are antioxidant, antiviral and antibacterial."[50]

Reishi is currently being used in combination with vitamin C to shrink human tumors. In Japan Fukumi Morishige, M.D., uses large doses of vitamin C to make polysaccharides more "bioavailable." In Thailand Dr. Santi Rosswong studies the same phenomenon, but he adds folic acid and caterpillar fungus to his tumor treatment.[51]

According to Dr. Clemmons, mushroom extracts stimulate a patient's immune system. They "present unique macromolecules to the intestinal tract, where they alter the immune regulation by intestinal antigen processing systems." Maitake mushroom extract has also been shown to activate NK killer cells (which attack tumor cells) and to halt the destruction of "good, T-Helper cells."[52]

One related supplement that can improve immune system function, writes Russell Swift, D.V.M., is MGN-3. This is a "blend of extracts from shiitake, kawaratake, and suehirotake mushrooms and rice bran," he explains. These extracts are "the leading prescription treatments for cancer in Japan." Studies on MGN-3 indicate that it can vastly increase natural killer-cell activity. He notes that these cells are necessary for the immune system.[53]

According to Dr. Raditic, while the ganoderma and gynostema mushrooms have "human formulas that we use for animals," the use of mushrooms in general in animal health is fairly new, without much related research.[54]

BACH FLOWER REMEDIES

Bach flower remedies were developed by Dr. Edward Bach (1880–1936), a physician from Mount Vernon, England. He found thirty-eight flowers that are ideal for use in healing negative emotional states. In 1930 he gave up his practice to devote all of his time to finding energies in the plant world that would restore vitality and enable patients to assist in their own healing processes.

The remedies are prepared from macerations of the flowers of wild plants, bushes, and trees in pure springwater that has been exposed to the sun for a few hours. None of them are harmful or addictive. The principle of the therapy is that the psychological aspects of illnesses and conditions are more important than the physical. Bach believed that a long-continued worry or fear will deplete an individual's vitality. By taking the appropriate remedy over time, peace and harmony can be achieved, allowing the body to produce its own natural healing.

Bach practiced what he preached. Occasionally he would suffer the negative state of mind for which a flower was needed, and at the same time he was what he termed "privileged" to suffer from some physical ailment. He would wander through fields at such times until he was "led" to the flowers that would restore his serenity and peace of mind. Within a few hours his physical complaint would also be healed.

The thirty-eight flowers are categorized under seven headings: those for anxiety and apprehension; for uncertainty and indecision; for loneliness; for insufficient interest in present circumstances; for oversensitivity to ideas and influence; for despondency and despair; and for overconcern for the welfare of others.

Bach Remedies are benign in action and produce no unpleasant reactions. More than one remedy may be taken at a time. The literature and instructions are self-explanatory. However, it is recommended that you not try to mix your own remedies, because these combinations of flowers are made following a special process. A dried herb concoction or infusion made at home will probably have no effect whatsoever.

Use in Animals

Several Bach remedies are given to animals today. Among the conditions treated with these mixtures are stress, shock, trauma, travel anxiety, jealousy of a new animal or human baby in the home, old age, aggression, and territorial behavior. One source for these products is PetSage Natural Remedies in Alexandria, Virginia. Like all responsible retailers and manufacturers, the company advises consulting your veterinarian first for recommendations of natural and alternative treatments.

Clare E. Middle, B.V.M.S., of Australia, often uses flower essences as part of a larger combination of modalities to treat small animals with cancer. She explains their use: "These treatments act at the outer auric or emotional levels as well as the physical to help resolve the ultimate psychic or emotional issue which has eventually become manifest as a physical disease." She believes it is "essential" that the disease be addressed at this level if a deep healing is to be possible.[55]

For example, Dr. Middle once treated a nine-year-old male rottweiler–German shepherd mix, Hagar Keay, for osteosarcoma of the left distal radius. The dog was diagnosed as a "mistake puppy" that used to be a boy's dog but during treatment lived with the boy's mother. When Middle first saw him, the dog was lame and depressed. He showed "fears at being left; [I used] flower essences for fear of rejection and resentment." The dog was treated in a variety of ways for four months; his tumor shrank and he became brighter and less lame for a time. Four months into the treatment, however, he slowly worsened and died. Explains Middle, "In retrospect, we could have kept up a higher dose of Essiac, and hands on psychic healing may have helped to remove the negative belief of the owner in 'terminal illness,' and the dog in feeling not totally loved. The flower essence treatment probably helped a lot in this regard." To be well treated, Middle feels that an animal with cancer needs a combination of therapies.[56]

Carolyn Ashton, B.V.Sc., also of Australia, has told me that she often uses flower essences. Although she states that she is loath to recommend specific amounts to administer, "as these are personal for the animals, e.g., dealing with fear, authority issues, letting go, etc.," she adds, "I would say, though, that Bach's Rescue Remedy (or equivalent) is general enough to apply to any situation."[57]

Dr. Middle tells of another veterinarian, Ian Gawler, who also runs a cancer retreat for people. His opinion is that many success stories of people who survive "incurable" cancers occur in the cases for which many treatments have been used. "The highest ranking of these treatments as judged by the patients themselves is recognizing and dealing with a major emotional or spiritual issue and changing to a natural and healthy diet," Middle states.[58]

Several veterinarians in the United States also believe in the calming benefits of flower essences for animals. Relates Stephen Blake, D.V.M., "We deal with a lot of emotions in animals. They grieve. They become angry. They do mischievous things to let us know they want more attention." He has practiced veterinary medicine for twenty-four years and finds that flower remedies are a simple and inexpensive way to help cure emotional problems and physical problems connected to them. Kymythy Schultze, a certified clinical nutritionist and animal health instructor who has written *Natural Nutrition for Dogs and Cats: The Ultimate Pet Diet,* uses Bach flower remedies, especially the five-essence combination known as Rescue Remedy or Five-Flower Formula. "No home should be without it," she says. "If shock or trauma is involved, always use Rescue Remedy first."

C. J. Puotinen, author of *The Encyclopedia of Natural Pet Care* and *Natural Remedies for Dogs and Cats,* finds that Bach flower remedies (BFR) work well and quickly in stressful, traumatic situations. She reports that they work well in combination with herbs, homeopathy, aromatherapy, and other natural remedies, as well as with pharmaceutical drugs. "They are nontoxic, don't affect the action of drugs, and are not affected by drugs."[59]

For weakness, exhaustion, chronic illness, or overall failing in a cat, Anita Frazier has often used BFR Formula IV. This consists of Wild Rose, Water Violet, Olive, Clematis, Sweet Chestnut, and Gorse. Her directions: Put two drops of each in a one-ounce dropper bottle. Fill to three-quarters full with springwater or distilled water, and shake the contents "vigorously" 108 times. Give your cat two or three drops every couple of hours. This remedy, says Frazier, will stay fresh in the refrigerator for two weeks. She says of Bach flower remedies overall, "the worst that will happen is nothing—zero results."[60]

Rita Reynolds, who has run an animal sanctuary in Virginia for more than twenty-five years, has always made use of whatever works to help her older and ailing animals become more comfortable and to feel less physical pain or abandonment issues. She primarily takes in elderly or unwanted dogs and cats. Although she has long used Rescue Remedy, she finds that recently it seems a bit weaker than in the past, and she heartily recommends a farm in New Hampshire, Green Hope Farm, which offers a beautiful and informative catalog of Bach flower remedies for people and other animals.[61]

Molly Sheehan, its founder, writes "Right now, animals are under a great deal of stress. The vibratory changes on Earth are particularly difficult for the animals. Most animals greatly need and appreciate Flower Essences. They dramatically ease an animal's burdens."[62] In February 2000, Green Hope Farm created a collection of twenty-two remedies called Animal Wellness Collection. All the farm's essences are stabilized in a base mixture of organic red shiso and a small amount of white vinegar. There are several remedies that would work well for an animal with cancer or one in the dying process, including: Abandonment & Abuse, Animal Emergency Care, Caretaker, Grief & Loss, Immune Support, Recovery, Senior Citizen, and Transition.

Some people have noted that these essences may take longer to take hold than prescribed Western medicine. Explained Sheehan, "If an animal does not respond in fairly short order, we usually have the human caretaker spritz the household with Essences mixed in water so that animals and people in the household are all getting the information of the Essences. This usually shifts the energy for the animal as everyone is now learning from the Essences."[63]

13 Vitamins and More

Animals need vitamins and minerals in proper amounts and ratios for ideal health. These vitamins and minerals help absorb fats and carbohydrates and are necessary for chemical reactions in the body. For example, if calcium and phosphorus are not in balance, it may lead to bone or muscle problems. Vitamins also are necessary for proper bone development. Many vitamins and minerals are contained in standard animal foods, but many are not there in adequate amounts. Supplementing a standard diet is encouraged by many veterinarians and nutritionists.

VITAMIN C

The vitamins you add to your dog's or cat's diet will depend on her health, size, and regular diet. Dogs manufacture their own vitamin C, but many veterinarians recommend adding more vitamin C for a variety of reasons, including to help treat or avoid some cancers and hip dysplasia, common in several breeds such as golden retrievers, German shepherds, and Labradors. Vitamin C seems to help with arthritis or muscular pain, and it is often given to dogs recovering from injury.

According to writer Catherine O'Driscoll, vitamin C is used to treat bladder cancer, mammary tumors, and cancer of the colon. Some vets are recommending it for patients who have just undergone surgery. Because it manufactures collagen within the body, it may also reduce the incidence of hip dysplasia. Wendell Belfield, an American veterinarian and author of several animal nutrition books, conducted an experiment on eight litters of German shepherd puppies from dysplastic parents (those who produce pups with dysplasia). These were given megadoses of vitamin C. The pregnant bitches were also given vitamin C. When the puppies were X-rayed at two years old, they were free of dysplasia.[1]

In another study, this one in Oslo, Norway, seventy-six dogs of various breeds and ages were given 30 milligrams of C-flex, a form of vitamin C, each day. All these dogs had some musculoskeletal condition such as joint injury, hip dysplasia, or muscle atrophy. After one week 76.3 percent showed good improvement or were free of symptoms. After six weeks this figure rose to 84.2 percent.

Vitamin C may protect against cancer because it acts as a cellular antioxidant. It enhances the immune system by detoxifying certain carcinogens and by blocking the formation of various carcinogenic compounds created when certain foods are digested. Several studies regarding nonhormone-dependent cancers in humans have suggested that this vitamin has a protective effect. It has also been shown to enhance the ability to survive infection in fish that had the vitamin added to their diets. In another animal-related study, supplementing poultry's diet with vitamin C appeared to enhance the birds' resistance to some bacterial and viral diseases.[2]

Author Pat Lazarus describes vitamin C's role this way: "Vitamin C increases the ability of white blood cells to get to, engulf, and destroy antigens; it also increases the production of Interferon."[3]

Because vitamin C is nontoxic, it cannot harm your dog if you give her too much, but a large amount of this vitamin can cause diarrhea in a dog. When you reduce the levels of the vitamin, the condition should stop. Catherine O'Driscoll recommends a daily supplement of vitamin C at the rate of approximately 50 to 100 milligrams per kilogram of dog's weight. She points to another veterinarian-author, Ian Billinghurst, who has said that a dog undergoing light stress could be fed 100 milligrams per kilogram; a dog moderately stressed, 200 milligrams per kilogram; heavily stressed, 300 milligrams per kilogram. Very heavily stressed dogs can be given 350 milligrams of vitamin C per kilogram of weight.[4]

Ann Martin, author of *Food Pets Die For,* also advocates additional vitamin C in animals' diets. She says that nutritional veterinarians have discovered that although dogs and cats do produce some vitamin C, stress, an illness, or an infection will deplete their natural supply. And as dogs age, their production of vitamin C decreases. She also points to Dr. Belfield, who recommends these dosages of vitamin C: for small dogs, 500 to 1,500 milligrams; medium-sized, 1,500 to 3,000 milligrams; large, 3,000 to 6,000 milligrams; and giant dogs, 6,000 to 7,500 milligrams. Her giant Newfoundland, Charlie, took about 3,000 milligrams of vitamin C a day in 1997 because he developed loose stools if she gave him more. She increased Charlie's dosage slowly and now uses powdered calcium ascorbate because it is easier on his stomach. She also recommends that if you give your dog a multivitamin and mineral supplement, you may wish to add more vitamin C.[5]

Richard Pitcairn, D.V.M., also recommends giving your pet vitamin C if you live in a particularly polluted area. This is especially useful to offset cadmium, lead, copper, and DDT, and he recommends zinc in this case, too. In this situation he would give between 100 and 500 milligrams of vitamin C and 5 to 20 milligrams of zinc, depending on the animal's size.[6]

Earl Mindell also recommends that all dogs take a daily supplement of vitamin C. He notes that Linus Pauling, the two-time Nobel prizewinner, discovered the important role that vitamin C plays in the prevention and the treatment of cancers.[7] In his last interview Pauling recalled two studies, one performed by Ewan Cameron, chief surgeon at Vale of Leven Hospital in Scotland, in which he gave 10 grams of vitamin C a day to patients with terminal cancer. Those who did not take the vitamin C lived an average of six months after they were labeled terminal; his C-ingesting patients lived an average of about six years more. In another study Pauling noted that the patients whom Abram Hoffer treated with about 12 grams of vitamin C a day lived about twelve years after being considered terminal with untreatable cancer. He did add that Hoffer's patients also received "eight hundred units of vitamin E, one thousand or two thousand milligrams of niacin, and large amounts of the other B vitamins and vitamin A in the form of beta carotene."

Pauling believed, at the end of his life, that every patient with cancer (this is human, remember) should take 10, 12, or more grams of vitamin C, 800 units of vitamin E, other vitamins, and 200 micrograms per day of selenium.[8]

Earl Mindell's recommended dosages of vitamin C are 500 to 1,000 milligrams for a small dog; 1,000 to 2,000 for a medium or large dog; and 2,000 to 4,000 for giant breeds.[9] His recommendations are more conservative than either Belfield's or Billinghurst's.

An even more conservative list was included in an article on vitamin C in the *1999 Annual Natural Cat* magazine. Based on extensive information from many veterinarians, author Liz Palika recommended for adult dogs (in tablets): small breeds, 250 milligrams; medium, 500; large, 750; and giant breeds, 1,000 milligrams. For adult cats, she recommended crushed tablets of 500 milligrams daily. These suggested dosages were all different if the animal was aging, ill, or injured, in which cases the dosage went up substantially.[10]

OTHER VITAMINS

Other recommended vitamins include some of the Bs, E, A, D, and K. The B vitamins help convert food to energy. The others are fat soluble and help in eyesight, bone formation, and strength (along with calcium), cell stability, and blood coagulation. A deficiency of vitamin E can cause reproductive failure and weakening of immune responses. Vitamin A deficiency can cause several eye problems, and deficiency of vitamin D can cause rickets. However, excessive vitamin A can lead to bone disease, and excessive vitamin D can cause hardening of soft tissue, lungs, and kidneys.[11]

Ann Martin also recommends vitamin E for dogs; it gave her dog Charlie "renewed vitality." Again quoting from Dr. Belfield that vitamin E "boosts the efficiency of the heart and the circulatory system," she follows his recommendation: for small dogs, 100 international units; medium dogs, 200 international units; large dogs, 200 international units; and giant dogs, 400 international units. She gave Charlie 200 international units in the form of d-alpha tocopherol. Martin is a firm believer in a natural diet and supplements. Charlie at that time was fourteen years old; the average life span of his breed is eight years.[12]

Regarding cats' needs, Martin writes that cats require more protein than dogs, thus more meat. They also require a lot of vitamin E, and because fish is low in this vitamin, too much fish is not a wise idea. She recommends purchasing a vitamin and mineral supplement at the pet food store to add to cats' diets, but she is not as specific about these additions as she is about the additions to the dogs' diets. Pitcairn explains in his book *Dr. Pitcairn's Complete Guide to Natural Health for Dogs and Cats* that cats cannot convert the beta-carotene in vegetables to vitamin A and thus they require it from an animal source such as cod-liver oil, cheese, or eggs. For felines he also recommends a preformed source of arachidonic acid (also in cod-liver oil) and taurine, an amino acid not found in plant foods. The latter is found in large concentrations in heart tissue and seafood and in smaller amounts in meats and dairy products. Pitcairn points to studies that show that a taurine-deficient diet can lead to blindness, heart problems, and other diseases in cats.[13]

Several studies have been performed regarding vitamin E's uses in animals' diets. It has been shown to stimulate the immune system in several animals when it is given at levels exceeding dietary requirements established for prevention of accepted clinical deficiency signs. In many studies performed between 1975 and 1984 of both laboratory and farm animals such as chicks, turkeys, lambs, calves, pigs, and mice, when their diets were supplemented with vitamin E, several things occurred: decreased mortality, increased weight, enhanced recovery, increased resistance, improved humoral immune response, and more. Writer Lawrence J. Machlin has concluded that vitamins E, C, and beta-carotene function as in-vivo antioxidants (which protect fats from becoming rancid-natural antioxidants including vitamins A, C, and E), and play an important role in slowing or even preventing "reduced immune function, cancer, cardiovascular disease, cataracts, arthritis, and dental disease in older animals."[14]

Martin's book on pet food includes a useful section on vitamins. I will list a few of her suggestions here, but I recommend her entire book if you would like an overview of what is really included in commercial pet foods and how you can wisely and lovingly improve your animal companion's diet.

Some of the foods that contain vitamin B_1 (thiamine) are beef liver and kidneys, whole grains, wheat germ, and kidney beans. Vitamin B_2 (riboflavin) may be found in cottage cheese, cheese, wheat germ, fish, chicken, and more. Vitamin B_3 (niacin) is found in beef liver, white chicken, peanuts, whole grains, and milk. Vitamin C can be found in oranges, peppers, broccoli, and most fruits and vegetables. Vitamin E is found in wheat germ, margarine, and eggs. This last vitamin is often used as a natural preservative in natural pet foods—for example, in California Natural dry foods.[15]

Vitamin K is also critical for dogs' diets; it aids in blood clotting and the production of protein and can most easily be found in liver or green vegetables.[16]

Vitamin A is found in fatty foods such as butter, cream, vegetable oil, and animal tissues, primarily liver. Carotinoids are found in bright yellow, orange-yellow, and dark green vegetables and are converted to vitamin A in the body. However, excess vitamin A can have a toxic effect. Symptoms may include swellings over long bones, dry or itchy skin, nausea and diarrhea, fatigue or lethargy, and loss of hair. Based on extensive research into vitamin A and ferrets' needs, writer Kathleen Cheeseman found that ferrets need approximately the same amount of vitamin A as minks (which have been studied for this nutritional requirement) on a daily basis—that is, 440 international units per pound for an adult. She believes that ferrets should be getting sufficient vitamin A from commercial foods but adds that no one has shown toxic effects in ferrets due to vitamin A. The species might have a deficiency situation rather than toxicity because of such conditions as shortsightedness and tooth staining.[17]

Robert McDowell, N.D., the herbalist from Australia, recommends vitamin C, which is abundantly found in fresh greens. He also offers this advice for a sick animal or one in shock: "A few Rosehips tea bags steeped in boiling water and allowed to cool will provide massive extra amounts of Vitamin C and Iron to aid in recovery."[18] He also recommends vitamin B: "Vitamin B_{12} is a specific cancer preventative and is best found in the herb Comfrey. This can be included occasionally and in small quantities in a green feed as a valuable supplement."[19]

CALCIUM

Calcium ranks high on the list of which minerals dogs and cats need in their diet. Pat Lazarus explains that calcium is essential for destroying foreign substances that are engulfed by white blood cells.[20]

One way to give your animals more calcium is to give them bones. Dr. Pitcairn includes bonemeal or another calcium supplement in the recipes in his books. He believes you can let your pet have bones occasionally, because they are the most natural source of calcium. However, he warns against chicken, turkey, fish, or pork bones, which splinter easily and can cause internal injuries; cooked bones are especially likely to splinter. He also cautions that if your dog is not used to eating bones, she may eat too much at one sitting at first, which could irritate her digestive tract. The dog could then either be constipated or have diarrhea. Also, for animals not in the greatest of health, digesting bones can be difficult. Pitcairn recommends going easy at first and limiting the time for your pet to chew on bones to a fifteen-minute trial period at the beginning.[21]

This issue of raw versus cooked bones—or any food item—has long been hotly debated among animal experts and nutritionists. Please refer back to chapter 7, Nutrition, for further discussion of the issue.

Earl Mindell, nutritionist and author of *Earl Mindell's Vitamin Bible,* recommends that dogs get their calcium in other forms. A few good sources are leafy green vegetables, soy, salmon, and nuts. Milk is not a good source, because it does not contain enough magnesium for the calcium to be used effectively.[22]

BETA-CAROTENE

Mindell feels that dogs at great risk for cancer should definitely take vitamin C, vitamin E, calcium, and two other supplements: beta-carotene and selenium. Beta-carotene reduces the risk of cancer and converts to vitamin A if a body needs that. It can be found in yellow, orange, and dark green vegetables and fruits or can be given with a vitamin E supplement, because they work together. If given in this form, Mindell recommends 15 international units for dogs of all sizes.

More than fifty studies in humans in the 1970s and 1980s correlated a high intake of foods high in beta-carotene with a reduced risk of certain cancers—lung, stomach, cervix, esophagus, throat, colon, breast, ovary, and mouth. The strongest correlations were with lung cancer. In other studies beta-carotene was shown to reverse precancerous lesions, especially oral ones. Several of the studies showed associations with specific foods rather than with the entire field of beta-carotene, but when blood levels of beta-carotene were measured, the association with a reduced risk of cancer was clear.[23]

SELENIUM

Selenium, an essential trace element, performs a variety of functions within the body, and one of those appears to help cancer patients. It is an antioxidant in the enzyme selenium-glutathione-peroxidase. It activates the enzyme gluathione peroxidase, which may protect the body against cancer. It also appears to stimulate antibody formation in response to vaccines. Selenium may provide some protection against heavy metal and other toxic substances and may also assist in the synthesis of protein and in growth and development. Generally taken as a mineral supplement or in a multivitamin, Earl Mindell suggests 25 micrograms for small dogs and 50 micrograms for all others.[24]

In a recent double-blind study of thirteen hundred people, those who ingested 200 micrograms of yeast-based selenium each day for seven years saw a 50 percent drop in the cancer death rate as compared to the placebo group.[25] Another human study looked at more than seven thousand men in Taiwan chronically infected with hepatitis B, hepatitis C, or both between 1988 and 1992. Sixty-nine of the men developed liver cancer during this period. The selenium levels were "significantly lower" in the cancer patients than in those who did not develop cancer. According to the scientists involved in the study at National Taiwan University in Taipei, earlier research had suggested that vitamin E and selenium supplements, taken together, resulted in a 13 percent reduction in cancer mortality in a study group that had high rates of cancers.[26]

According to Joel Wallach, D.V.M., more than one hundred animal studies have shown that giving animals diets rich in selenium may help protect them against breast, esophagus, and liver cancers. Selenium is naturally found in high-protein foods: fish, meat, poultry, cereals, and grains. Mushrooms and asparagus also contain high levels of the substance.[27]

Pat Lazarus quotes Dr. Martin Goldstein's selenium recommendations: 50 to 100 micrograms daily at mealtimes. Please note that this amount is *not* 50 or 100 *milligrams,* a much higher amount that could cause harm.[28] Susan G. Wynn, D.V.M., notes that selenium may also reduce chemotherapy's adverse effects.[29]

However, not everyone is so confident about this mineral's anti-cancer qualities. In a 1996 article in the Journal of the American Medical Association, a dozen writers say that "selenium CAN prevent cancer. Unfortunately, you would need to take a lethal dose of selenium." They point out that earlier studies had connected selenium with a slight decrease in lung, prostate, and colorectal cancers, but not with any other cancers. They also point out that selenium was only "WEAKLY" associated with a decrease in incidence of cancer. These authors advise taking all studies with a grain of salt, and they advise, in a lighthearted tone, that selenium is definitely good for one thing: "It's the active ingredient in dandruff shampoo."[30]

Dr. Wynn also recommends these possible supplements: coenzyme Q10 (which is immune enhancing and may "reduce toxicity of the chemotherapeutic drug adriamycin"), arginine, pycnogenol, melatonin (which suppresses some cancer types), and glandulars—especially extracts of thymus gland, which "may contain cytokines helpful in managing cancer."[31]

14 Homeopathy and Naturopathy

Both homeopathy and naturopathy are treatment practices with philosophies that consider health holistically, taking into account that people and animals are made up of both physical and emotional components, and that illness may affect a number of these components at the same time. Those who treat animals using either of these two modalities believe that at the root of health is an innate, instinctive life force or energy, and that animals have a natural capacity and ability to heal.

HOMEOPATHY

Although considered modern by many, homeopathy dates as far back as Hippocrates, the father of medicine. The system being used today was developed in Germany by Samuel Christian Hahnemann, a medical doctor in the mid-1800s.

Kaetheryn Walker, author of *Homeopathic First Aid for Animals,* explains its philosophical basis this way: "Homeopathy is based on the Law of Similars, which states that 'like cures like.'. . . Simply put, a substance that causes symptoms when given in a large amount to a healthy individual will also cure similar symptoms when given in minute amounts to an ill individual . . . they stimulate the natural immune system to mount a defense, which results in a momentum building toward the health of the organism."[1]

Homeopathic medicines are prepared with substances from the animal, vegetable, and mineral kingdoms. Plants are harvested in their natural habitat by specialists, and brought in their fresh form for laboratory conversion. Venoms, hormones, and organs of animals are used for extracts. Mineral salts and metals are treated in the laboratory. A preparation known as the mother tincture results from the maceration of plants and other base products in alcohol. This tincture is the initial source, and it is diluted for the preparation of a given homeopathic medication into infinitesimal doses. The tradition is to use minute doses of a substance that will provoke desired symptoms in a healthy individual to heal the same symptoms in an ill individual—like cures like. Homeopathy deals with the whole person or animal and with any psychological barriers.

Homeopathic medications come in granules, doses, globules, or drops. Drops are generally taken before meals with water. Each is administered by placing under the tongue, where it dissolves. Homeopathic medication should not be touched with the fingers because its surface is active. It is meant to be poured directly into the mouth from the capsule in which it is contained.

Some skeptics point out that homeopathy's tenets lack serious scientific study; much of its reputation relies on anecdotal evidence, because major institutions do not invest in huge studies in this treatment. And indeed, the use of homeopathy requires a leap of faith, as well as deep trust between the doctor and the patient and (in the case of animals) the patient's human companion. It requires suspending distrust of new methods and putting aside familiar ones that have been trusted over an entire lifetime.

Homeopathy is now used quite widely with small animals, and quite often for treating cancer. The (initial) certification program for homeopathic veterinary medicine takes place over a year and includes education, experiential work, presentation of papers, and supervised work.

One of its most famous practitioners in the United States and one of the most respected is Richard Pitcairn, D.V.M., author of several books and a teacher of postgraduate courses in veterinary homeopathic techniques. He has told me, "Gradually we are training veterinarians in methods of healing instead of suppression." He runs the Animal Natural Health Center in Eugene, Oregon, and established the

Academy of Veterinary Homeopathy. Although Dr. Pitcairn uses dietary changes, Bach flower remedies, and homeopathic remedies and mixtures for his patients with cancer, he says, "My primary focus is the use of homeopathy, not [on treating] cancer, though I end up treating some of these cases. Most are not cured in my hands."[2]

Russell Swift, D.V.M., says this about cancer and homeopathy: "There is a myriad of other so-called anti-cancer products available. Before going beyond the above recommendations [diet, vaccines, water, and so on], I would suggest contacting a qualified homeopath. Homeopathy can get to the deeper levels of the disease process. This is where the ultimate cure resides."[3]

One of the frustrations for veterinarians who employ these methods is that they often see the animals when they are on their last legs, rather than throughout their entire lives or at the onset of the disease. If conventional methods of treatment have not worked, animal guardians may turn to a homeopathic veterinarian.

For this book, I interviewed George Glanzberg, V.M.D., of North Bennington, Vermont. Glanzberg has been trained in homeopathic practices by Dr. Pitcairn. I found him through a kind and thorough article he had written for an alternative newspaper in southern Vermont. "We believe that good health comes essentially from within the animal's own body," he writes. "Good health is based on maintaining the body in a way that promotes its natural healing capacity."[4]

A veterinarian for thirty years, Dr. Glanzberg has combined conventional and homeopathic medicine in his small animal practice in Vermont for twenty years. He does perform surgery and give routine vaccines but prefers to treat dogs and cats homeopathically, working with natural diets and more. The acceptance of these methods is improving in his geographical area. Approximately one-third to one-half of his clients choose to have their animals treated homeopathically. Patients come to him from both New York and Vermont, some driving 150 miles one way to avail themselves of his services.

When a client agrees to treat his or her animal with an alternative medical procedure, Dr. Glanzberg needs to first gather information about the animal's personality and life. He spends an hour with the animal to obtain a detailed assessment. Both physical and emotional factors are considered. "I give the dog a cookie, play with it, take a walk with it. I ask why the owner is here and explain to the owner I need to know more. We talk about the inception of their relationship, the animal's personality, its likes and dislikes, its maladies. Then I examine the dog and play with it some more. We will talk about nutrition, and in many cases, I may want to do more diagnostic work, for example, X-rays," he explains.

But an X-ray is about as far as he wants to go in most cases. He also performs blood work, cardiograms, and other noninvasive procedures. Dr. Glanzberg is conservative and cautious about performing a biopsy, standard treatment among conventional veterinarians. "Every biopsy comes at a price to the animal. It may not get an appropriate tissue or it may puncture an unwanted hole. I'm often torn about what to do. I feel my way with every case. Cancer is not an overall disease; each one is almost its own disease."

He defines the difference between conventional cancer treatment and homeopathic treatment like this: "In homeopathy, we really mean cure. We're working with the body's own resources. The body has the capacity to actually cure. Or we can palliate [alleviate or mitigate, not cure] with homeopathy. I always ask, can I cure or palliate this case? In cancer cases, it's not unusual to make the choice to palliate."

He continues, "In many cases, we have done as well with no surgery, radiation, or chemotherapy. The animal has lived as long, undoubtedly leading a happier, healthier life."[5]

There are a number of success stories of Dr. Glanzberg treating animals with cancer. In August 1995 an older dog had a mammary tumor removed. The dog also had a bloated stomach, was severely arthritic, and was on two medications. Dr. Glanzberg put him on a natural food diet and treated him homeopathically. His tumors began to shrink but then regrew. The veterinarian changed the remedies and removed a tumor in July 1998. Now, six years into treatment, the dog has no masses and is still relatively healthy.

A cat born in 1984 had an enlarged kidney, diagnosed in 1994. The cat had high total protein and high calcium. He probably had cancer of the kidney. "He was vomiting, emaciated, and tired," explains the veterinarian. Dr. Glanzberg didn't biopsy the kidney but treated it homeopathically. The cat underwent no surgery and is still alive and being treated homeopathically.

Like many holistic veterinarians, Dr. Glanzberg advocates a natural, home-cooked diet for all animal companions (he follows Dr. Pitcairn's advice and hands out recipes to patients' caregivers) and believes the use of chemicals—on lawns, on gardens, and in commercial flea products—contributes to many chronic medical conditions in animals today. He does not believe in excessive vaccinations, adding that "a modest amount is important, for example, for rabies." He notes that it is extremely important to minimize exposure to pollutants and toxins and, overall, to maintain as healthy a lifestyle as possible for your animals.[6]

Half the world away in western Australia, Dr. Clare E. Middle uses many holistic treatments for cancer. In the past five years she has treated approximately seventy small animals in a variety of ways. These were animals "for which there was no suitable conventional therapy," she explains. She uses a variety of techniques including homeopathy, acupuncture, flower essences, and herbs. Regarding homeopathy, she says, "Many classical homeopaths happily and successfully treat cancer using homeopathy only, as many ting point [points at the tips of the toes and fingers] acupuncturists do likewise with ting points, but I find a greater success using thoughtful combinations."[7]

Another Australian natural animal healer, who has worked with animals since the mid-1980s and been in clinical practice since 1992, is Kathleen Griffin, N.D. (qualified naturopath), of the Natural Therapy Centre for Animals. She explains the therapy this way: "Homeopathy is a very useful form of medicine to assist a being to achieve a state of grace in a certain situation because high potency homeopathy is able to alter the inheritance, the genetic code, or the programming that an animal has brought into this lifetime in its genetic code."[8]

She relates the case study of Vaska, a malamute for whom several homeopathic remedies worked remarkably well. Vaska has been raised on a natural diet of raw meat, vegetables, whole grains, and meaty bones. He lives with Helen Spivak, a breeder and shower of malamutes, who wanted his story to be told.

Once, when she was overseas on holiday, Spivak returned to find Vaska much thinner. He also behaved differently; he did not want to go inside. Spivak took Vaska to a conventional veterinarian, who initially diagnosed his condition as a viral infection. A blood test showed that

Vaska was low in protein, and his white blood count was "raided." Although the veterinarian advised antibiotics and a diet of Eukanuba, Spivak refused these options; Vaska had been given natural nutrition and medicines for all his five and a half years. The dog continued to lose weight and quite suddenly lost the use of his back legs. After a chiropractic treatment, Vaska was placed on an anti-inflammatory medicine. His condition seemed to improve, but he continued to lose weight. Spivak then consulted a holistic veterinarian, who, during palpation, found what appeared to be a very enlarged liver. An ultrasound showed nothing. The veterinarian "pronounced a liver infection and a biopsy and antibiotic therapy," explains Griffin. Spivak began vitamin and mineral therapy for the dog, giving Vaska large doses of B-complex and C vitamins.

The malamute had a further blood test, which showed that his blood protein was still low and his white cell count raised. The holistic veterinarian, Dr. Ann Neville of Melbourne, performed a needle aspirate. She found *E. coli,* thought to be coming from the liver but ultimately discovered to be coming from the duodenum. They decided to operate on Vaska and found an enormous mass the size of a football in his stomach. This occurred in November 1997. Although one option was to put the dog to sleep, his guardian refused this. After consulting several holistic animal therapy books, she ordered laetrile from New Zealand. Dr. Neville agreed to perform intravenous vitamin C therapy on the dog.

After three days of this therapy Vaska's stomach seemed to decrease in size. Within three weeks the dog appeared to be quite healthy. Spivak continued this nutritional therapy for several months.

Kathleen Griffin first saw Vaska as a patient in September 1998. Although the dog seemed to have recovered from his bout with cancer, he still had a smell to his coat, and she tested his energy field pattern with the Vegatest system, an electroacupuncture diagnostic device. Griffin used deep homeopathic medicines (Thuja LM1) to "clear the hereditary and karmic predisposition to cancer from his genetic coding," and herbal remedies and hands-on energy balancing for his liver and heart. As of February 2000 Vaska was still well, had regained weight and energy, and was a happy dog.[9]

Dr. Carolyn Ashton, also of Australia, uses homeopathic and other natural approaches alone or after the animal has had radical surgery. She appreciates it when her clients are drawn to natural approaches. She cites this example: Two families with dogs diagnosed with cancer "were already interested in natural therapies and didn't just grab at these as a lifeline. . . . Interestingly enough, neither of [the dogs] were 'cured' in the sense that the word is often used, although you'd have to agree that they had a great and precious extension to their life."[10]

Based in Villars en Pons, France, Anna Guitton, D.V.M., has been using homeopathy and other alternative therapies since 1982. She runs seminars and workshops on animal communication "to animal owners who already have an openness to it." She has told me about one case in which she used homeopathy to extend a comfortable life. A seven-year-old golden retriever had liver and pancreas cancer. Following abdominal explorative surgery, he lived comfortably for one and a half years after this diagnosis was made. Dr. Guitton gave him homeopathic remedies, a homemade diet (she always checks the diet before making any other recommendations for treatment), various food supplements, and a little organtherapy. Derived from homeopathy, this therapy uses body parts or secretions, such as pancreas or kidney tissue, in microscopic quantities; they are generally used for the long-term rebuilding of the same organ in the patient or for boosting the particular function. She saw him each month and used no standard medicine except for the vitamins. Homeopathy even helped him die. He declined rapidly at the end, and a homeopathic remedy helped him pass away smoothly. "No shot was necessary," says Guitton. "He died peacefully at home."[11]

NATUROPATHY

Animal naturopathy, like homeopathy, considers the whole animal—both physical and emotional. Its preventive approach attempts to make the body's natural healing ability stronger. Treatments include the use of herbs, vitamins, minerals, essences, natural nutrition, homeopathy, energy balancing, and human-animal communications. Stress management and exercise therapy may also be used, sometimes in combination with standard medical therapies.

According to definitions from the General Council and Register of Naturopaths, a governing and registering body of qualified naturopaths in the United Kingdom, naturopathic medicine is quite ancient, with its philosophical basis and many of its methods dating back at least as far as Hippocrates. Naturopathic medicine's philosophy rests on three basic principles. The first is that the body possesses the ability to heal itself through internal vitality and intelligence. The second is that disease equals a manifestation of this vital life force "applying itself to the removal of obstructions to the normal functioning of organs and tissues." The basic causes of disease are chemical (imbalances in the body's chemistry), mechanical (muscular tensions, stiff joints, and other interferences to movement), and psychological (often caused by stress). The third principle is that naturopathic medicine embodies a holistic approach to healing. "The naturopathic practitioner searches for causes at many levels, and attempts to eliminate the fundamental cause of illness, not simply to remove symptoms."[12]

According to practitioners at the Natural Therapy Centre for Animals in Melbourne, Australia, "Naturopathic philosophy recognises all living creatures as having an inherent 'life-force' or energy which is the basis of health." Sometimes the life force becomes weakened— physically, mentally, emotionally, or spiritually—because of bad diet, toxic substances, grief, or trauma. Then the body may develop disease. Naturopathy can help restore the primary life force with gentle medicines and healing techniques. Like many alternative veterinarians, animal naturopaths attempt to prevent disease by increasing health and energy through diet and other holistic methods of care before the onset of illness.[13]

Practitioners at the Killarney Cat Hospital in Calgary, Canada, explain naturopathy in this way: "In the last decade, naturopathy has seen a new resurgence in popularity. Naturopathy views the animal being as a complete entity encompassing all levels of existence . . . all integrally intertwined and independent, making up the whole animal." The cats that are treated at this hospital receive a combination of Western and complementary or alternative medicine.[14]

Richard Pitcairn, D.V.M., explains that naturopaths believe the major physical cause of disease is a buildup of toxic materials in the body—often associated with poor eating and insufficient exercise. Naturopaths believe that toxic materials close the usual routes to disposing of waste. Some methods naturopaths employ with their patients may be fasting, drinking pure water or juices, taking enemas, hot and cold treatments, sunbathing, adopting a new nutritious diet, and more. Dr. Pitcairn does not recommend fasting for an animal with a "wasting disease" such as cancer.[15]

Almost any condition can benefit from some form of natural healing, believes Kathleen Griffin. She has told me that conditions for which naturopathy has been especially successful include cystitis and hyperactivity in cats, skin problems and arthritis in dogs, and lameness and personality problems in horses. She explains her philosophy: "We do not treat disease, we treat the whole animal. Obviously nutritional assistance is beneficial. We use homeopathics to clear the heredity miasms and karma and also to relieve symptoms and tone, strengthen and balance the body; herbal remedies are also beneficial, both nutritionally and for their etheric [subtle energy field] vibrations, and flower essences are a must. The most important aspect of an animal's healing is their mind. If they feel good, at peace, they will be good!"[16]

Dr. Pitcairn also believes that naturopathy can effectively be used with other alternative or holistic approaches, such as herbs, chiropractic, acupuncture, traditional Chinese medicine, and homeopathy.[17]

One extremely ill cat under naturopathic care proved to be an absolute success story. The cat had inflammatory bowel disease and was given a poor prognosis. Dinah was put on Hill's Prescription Diet w/d and on prednisone. She continued on this regimen for four years and had occasional recurrences of the disease. Then the cat's new veterinarian, Jeff Feinman of Connecticut, told the family of naturopathic treatment, and they began to read all they could. With the doctor's guidance, they switched all four of their cats to a homemade diet: lamb or turkey, with brown rice or potatoes, squash, and some clover sprouts. They gave Dinah additional herbal remedies such as apple pectin and liquid chlorophyll, along with slippery elm syrup before each meal. She went from being a listless cat to an active one; she lost the weight she had gained on her former regimen; her coat improved. "What is so ironic in this was our recent discovery that the 'cure' we were instructed to give her, the corticosteroid treatments, may have contributed to the long-term worsening of her disease and her general health." The guardians now suspect that the disease may have begun as an allergic response. Their cats are now all healthy.[18]

One successful U.K. naturopathic pet care business, Denes Natural Pet Care, was begun in 1951 by Buster Lloyd-Jones, a veterinary surgeon who practiced for many years in the Brighton-Hove area of England. He did not actually qualify as a vet; wartime service prevented him from completing his formal studies. But he practiced veterinary medicine for approximately thirty-five years, up until his death in 1980. Among his clients were Winston Churchill's dogs.[19]

Lloyd-Jones is still considered a pioneer in the use of herbal remedies and natural foods for cats and dogs. He noticed during his lifetime, much of it spent in a wheelchair and, later, in bed due to polio, that his own animal companions liked to eat wild herbs and berries. He learned from observing them that they were following their instincts to find natural remedies for various conditions (much the way John Hoxsey's horse had found a natural remedy for his growths; see chapter 12, Herbs and Bach Flower Remedies).

In *Come into My World: Animals and Other People*, his second book, first published in 1972, Lloyd-Jones writes, "Those were the days before penicillin, of course, and there was nothing like the complexity of drugs available as there is now."[20] He believes he was the only homeopathic vet practicing in his region; he preferred traditional remedies, including "aconite, belladonna, nux vomica, and digitalis," but also used conventional drugs "in extreme cases." But the drugs were hard to come by—as was nutritious food—during World War II. "The bombed-out and evacuated dogs in my care had to eat, but people had priority over animals and food too was scarce." So he turned to nature for the answers. "I fed the animals as much as possible on home-grown produce. They ate greens, onions and even root vegetables for bulk." He notes that wartime diets were not great for people either. Lloyd-Jones discovered at this time that dogs with gastric conditions or worms responded well to garlic and sought it out themselves. He crushed it in a mortar and pestle and made many experiments as to its quantity. Often his results "were spectacular."[21]

Throughout the entire war he experimented with natural ingredients, keeping tables and charts. "It was all very promising and when peace came I began to think I was really getting somewhere." He approached a well-known group of London herbalists to ask them to make powders and pills from natural ingredients. His first Denes

Veterinary Herbal Products were garlic pills, seaweed powder, elderberry pills, and greenleaf pills, made from the chlorophyll of various leaves and herbs.[22]

The veterinarian also relates this story in his charming second memoir. He once treated a lovely bitch with impressive breeding—Laurette, a poodle who lived in Paris with the Goldschmidt-Halot family. The dog was suffering from malnutrition at the least, as were many people at that time. Lloyd-Jones brought along no drugs, but decided he could select natural medicines from the countryside to treat her. He took the couple out to Neuilly and showed them what herbs to give Laurette. The couple were so happy with his advice they asked him to create a small descriptive catalog for them, listing the herbs and their uses. The Goldschmidt-Halots treated not only their dog but also dozens of children with his natural remedies. Laurette began to recover her good health almost immediately.[23]

Denes Natural Pet Care now carries a wide range of foods, herbal medicine, supplements, and aromatherapy products for both dogs and cats. Its products contain no artificial colors, flavors, or preservatives, and all are free of soy. The company adds herbs such as parsley, thyme, and dandelion for flavor, aroma, and essential vitamins and minerals. The firm is located in Hove, East Sussex, and the products are sold in the United Kingdom; some are available by mail order. See the resources in the back of this book for more information. Unfortunately, they are still not available in the United States. Writes Peter Leaney, managing director of Denes, "In the past we have approached the FDA and the CVM (Committee for Veterinary Medicine) with details of our products, many of which are licensed herbal veterinary medicines here in the UK." However, they are still unable to export to the United States. The company does export its products to Japan and to the Netherlands.[24]

15 Other Alternative Therapies

Many other alternative therapies exist to complement any of those previously mentioned or any conventional treatments you and your veterinarian decide are best for your animal who has been diagnosed with cancer. In addition, the following modalities, along with homeopathy and naturopathy, herbal and Bach flower remedies, and vitamin therapy, can be used as part of a holistic treatment plan for a number of other illnesses or conditions your animal may be facing.

ACUPUNCTURE

Acupuncture—the application of small-gauge needles to precise points in the body for treatment of many ailments and conditions and relief of pain—is an ancient procedure used originally in traditional Chinese medicine. A primitive acupuncture therapy was practiced in India approximately seven thousand years ago. The classical explanation of the Chinese technique is that energy channels run in patterns through the body and over its surface. The basic tenet of traditional Chinese medicine holds that vital life energy, called qi or chi, flows through the body in these channels or meridians. But the channels can become obstructed, and any obstruction or blockage can eventually lead to disease.[1]

According to David J. Gilchrist, B.V.Sc., veterinary surgeon and acupuncturist in Australia, "Acupuncture points, which lie on the meridians, are areas of the skin . . . at which the flow of 'chi' [energy] can be influenced." When a person or animal is diseased, an imbalance exists in the flow of energy. A skilled acupuncturist, by stimulating these points, can manipulate the flow of energy and thus remedy the imbalance.[2]

The earliest reference to acupuncture's use in humans in America appeared in a medical journal of 1836, but the procedure did not make its way into the *New England Journal of Medicine* until 1926. Those early references were positive; by the 1980s many Western veterinary and medical establishments were regularly using acupuncture as a tool. Today nearly three million veterinary practitioners, assistants, and pharmacists are trained in the techniques. The International Veterinary Acupuncture Society (IVAS) of Longmont, Colorado, includes most of them as members, maintains a Web site, and publishes a journal.[3]

But using these techniques on nonhumans is not brand new. According to David Gilchrist, acupuncture has been used for animals for thousands of years. "Western scientists are still undecided how it works, although they agree that it does," Dr. Gilchrist notes. The acupuncture diagnosis revolves around knowing what area of the body has a problem. Treatment with acupuncture requires a knowledge of "what meridians pass through that area; what points on that meridian should be stimulated; what method of stimulation should be used; and what other special points on other meridians will have a beneficial effect on the problem." Although most acupuncturists use the traditional needles, some now also use laser beams. Gilchrist feels that the laser beam "has revolutionized the practice of acupuncture" because it is painless, it is easier to perform, it cannot introduce infection, it takes less time, and it is relatively cheap. Treatment with a special helium-neon laser is safe for tissue, and the newest infrared lasers are also safe when used correctly. Electro-acupuncture can be used in cases when needles or lasers do not seem effective.[4]

Although these techniques are gaining popularity in the United States, they are perhaps more widespread in Europe and Australia. Especially in France and parts of Scandinavia, acupuncture is routinely used to treat animals with various conditions, including cancer. Edward J. Boldt Jr., D.V.M., is the executive director of IVAS; he notes that the group currently has approximately 1250 members, most all of whom are certified. The bulk of the members live in the United States, but as it is an international organization, they have members worldwide. "We have more members in Australia than we do in Canada," he told me. "Veterinary acupuncture continues to grow around the world," says Dr. Boldt. "We continue to see more practices offering veterinary acupuncture to their clients, as well as more universities showing interest. Veterinary acupuncture continues to grow as more pet owners look to complementary medicine for their own health care, they look for veterinarians to offer it to their pets."[5]

To become certified, a licensed veterinarian in good standing must attend courses in basic veterinary acupuncture theory and skills, take exams, and submit case reports or perform an internship. Certification is awarded a minimum of one year following graduation from a veterinary college. (This time period may be extended in some countries.) The IVAS Basic Course, taught in the United States, accepts one hundred new veterinarians each year.[6]

One example of a veterinarian who has been successful using acupuncture is Are Thoresen, D.V.M., of Sandefjord, Norway. Dr. Thoresen became a conventional veterinarian in 1979 and has also trained as a homeopath. He studied acupuncture in France and Finland and was officially certified in 1981 for humans and 1989 for animals. He notes that acupuncture and other alternative methods are popular in Norway and elsewhere. "Here and in France, perhaps 30 to 40 percent of animals are partly or mainly treated with alternative methods, usually acupuncture."[7] Most acupuncture is done on horses and on dogs, although Thoresen does sometimes treat cats as well.

Thoresen has had much success treating cancer with acupuncture, especially mammary cancer. His first case involved this condition. "I tried a special method in my neighbor's dog. He was about eight years old and the mammary cancer was spreading to the lungs. I treated it twice and it all disappeared. The dog never had surgery and lived for five years." Usually, Thoresen treats the animal one to three times. He administers one treatment, waits fourteen days and administers a second; then waits perhaps a month before giving a third treatment. He claims to an 80 percent healing rate in mammary tumors in dogs (and also in women) whether they have had surgery or not. He has successfully treated at least 150 dogs and many horses.[8]

His method is to focus on only one point, though he may use up to three command points (special points on the twelve main meridians). "In cancer therapy it is of crucial importance to use only ONE point. . . . The point should control the cancer."[9]

Thorsen explains, "The Americans use more needles, but fewer needles have a better effect. It's like dealing with a disobedient child. You say only one thing and that's very powerful." Besides treating mammary cancer, he has also had success with brain, skin, and uterine cancer. Liver cancer is more difficult to treat. Nevertheless, he continues, "In almost 100 percent of my cases, acupuncture has had an effect. The appetite is better; the light in their eyes is better. Acupuncture works in healing, but sometimes, of course, the treatment is too late." Even then, however, he can still raise the qi. In this case the animal may live for one day, several days, or even several months; she will "gain weight and happiness. If the treatment is not too late, I can cure the cancer. The cancer disappears although there might be a connective tissue lump remaining."[10]

Mary L. Brennan, D.V.M., a holistic veterinarian in Georgia, has used Thoresen's cancer treatment in her acupuncture practice. She writes that his method "is not effective 100 percent of the time, but many complex forms of cancer have responded to treatment and I have found it very valuable."[11]

An alternative view of acupuncture for animals, this from a human doctor, comes from Andrew Weil, M.D. He reiterates the possible use of acupuncture in animals for a variety of ailments: arthritis, dysplasia, epilepsy, immune system suppression, and more. However, he points out cautiously, "This treatment has not been used for cancer in humans, though, and it's never been represented as a cancer treatment. It is, however, very helpful for pain reduction." As do most doctors, human and animal, Dr. Weil recommends choosing wisely when you look for an acupuncturist. "Make sure that person has been trained in animal acupuncture and not just on humans. . . . You may also want to try some acupressure on your own. I'm sure a loving massage by you could do wonders to relieve your dog's pain."

Like many alternative doctors, Dr. Weil recommends veterinarian Cheryl Schwartz's *Four Paws Five Directions: A Complete Guide to Traditional Chinese Medicine for Dogs and Cats*, for background, advice, and step-by-step daily directions for massages for your pet.[12]

According to another doctor of humans, Raymond Chang, M.D.,

several well-documented studies have shown acupuncture to be an excellent preventive measure against the nausea and vomiting associated with chemotherapy (and, incidentally, with pregnancy).[13]

For more information or to find a veterinarian trained in the use of acupuncture in your area, contact IVAS (see the resources at the end of this book). This group holds courses and international conferences, promotes research, and maintains a list of members accredited for training and instruction in veterinary acupuncture practices.

THE TELLINGTON TTOUCH

The Tellington TTouch is a massage technique introduced by Linda Tellington-Jones that reduces tension and changes behavior in dogs and other animals. It is often used with aggressive, timid, or sore animals. Tellington-Jones, a horse trainer and competitive rider, author of *The Tellington TTouch* and *Improve Your Horse's Well-Being*, developed a method of circular touches, similar to body awareness exercises developed for humans by Moshe Feldenkrais, to enhance her traditional training methods.

The central TTouch motion is made in the shape of a circle. Place your fingertips on the animal's body and trace a clock-face circle from six o'clock around the dial past the starting point to eight o'clock. The pressure, speed, and size of the motion depend on the animal. Circles are traced all over the body with one or two fingers, including on the face and even on the gums. There are many variations on circles, such as slides, and rubs; even the ear can be rubbed in a sliding motion from base to tip. An overall body rub can also be given.

According to veterinarian Tom Beckett and his assistant TTeam practitioner, Marnie Reeder, "The circular TTouch elicits changes in brain wave patterns . . . human and animal relate as two autonomous thinking creatures with increased self-confidence, enhanced communications, and mutual respect. . . . TTeam does not change the animal's basic nature, . . . and it does not use force, fear or pain." This technique is used as an enhancement of, not as a replacement for, traditional medical techniques.[14]

The technique relies on both bodywork and groundwork. The bodywork consists of specific touches to treat both physical and emotional problems. The groundwork involves guiding the animal through exercises that result in her moving "in nonhabitual ways." The two are designed to calm the animal, to create a relaxed, attentive state of being, and to bring out feelings.

The process is relatively easy to perform and it takes little time to achieve results. Training involves three one-hour sessions, held one week apart.[15]

The TTouch philosophy includes such statements as "to honor the role of animals as our teachers; to respect each animal as an individual; [and] to teach interspecies communication through the TTouch." The therapy has an educational organization, Animal Ambassadors International, dedicated to sharing the philosophy and techniques to "heal our relationships with others, nature and the environment."[16]

Tellington TTouch was used with one golden retriever, Alexandra of the Cincinnati area, who was uncomfortable following surgical removal of a lump on the right side of her chest. The mass, after being evaluated, was found to be a well-differentiated chondrosarcoma, a malignant tumor of cartilage that can sometimes become invasive. However, the fact that this tumor was well differentiated indicated it might not spread much.

A month later chest X-rays showed no spread to the lungs, but Alexandra was back in the clinic the following month with weakness in her front legs. She did not want to climb stairs. Her veterinarian treated Alex with low-dose steroids, and she was well for two more months. Then the tumor returned to the previous site. Her prognosis was only a few months, and Alex's owner, Barbara, agreed to keep her comfortable and allow her to enjoy her remaining time. Barbara then saw Dr. April Linville, who recommended vitamins and holistic remedies, and advised the owner to contact Susan Spalter, a registered TTouch practitioner who lived in their area.

Writes Susan Spalter, "The first session involved certain touches to help calm Alex and Barbara. . . . All agreed that Alex arrived as a tired, somewhat anxious dog and left more relaxed with that typical Golden smile." The dog grew more at ease and woke up more refreshed and more interested in her daily life. "Alex soon learned to nudge Barbara when she came home from work—to let her know it was time for the touches," notes Spalter.

Unfortunately, the tumor continued to grow quite quickly, and in about a month's time Alexandra was put to sleep. However, Barbara said this: "TTouch reinforced the bond between Alex and me. . . . Every morning she was ready and waiting for her peanut butter and pills and every evening she was ready for a good TTouch session. It reduced stress for Alex and for me."[17]

Another story illustrating the use of TTouch comes from author and publisher Rita Reynolds, who always has about twenty-five animals of various ages and conditions living in her Virginia home. One of these was Waggy, a mixed-breed ten-year-old dog with cancer of the mouth. Following surgery the cancer went into remission, but within a year it had returned. Writes Reynolds, "Waggy came and told me when it was time to help her out of her pain. It was still hard, because she had eaten breakfast that morning, and walked to the car." In the car she sat up straight in the front seat and looked out the window, as she had always done. But her message had been clear: "She was ready to go on."

When they arrived at the animal hospital, Waggy became frightened, as animals often do. Reynolds had to carry her in. Because the dog weighed about sixty pounds, this was not an easy task. Waggy began to panic in the exam room as they waited for the doctor.

"I talked to her and tried to calm her down, but I was fighting tears myself, and so I wasn't much help." Then Reynolds thought of TTouch. "I began doing large circles all over her body. By breathing into the circles, as Tellington-Jones recommends, and focusing on the process, I was able to stop my own mind from the runaway emotions I had begun to have and Waggy, in turn, began to relax." Reynolds at first paced her own breathing with Waggy's rapid pace, then began to slow hers down. Waggy's also slowed.

"By the time the doctor came into the room," recalls Reynolds, "and she was given the shot, she was completely relaxed, as was I, and she eased peacefully on. Doing the TTouch definitely helped."[18]

Reynolds has also used the TTouch techniques on two of her donkeys, Nori and Miso. The first case involved a digestive crisis, and the second, sarcoids (benign external tumors that bleed). Miso, age twelve, had developed a sarcoid at the base of his ear. It grew and bled until it was the size of a grapefruit. The donkey did not want Reynolds to touch the sarcoid or any other part of his body. Although Reynolds wanted to clean the dried blood off his face and put something on the sarcoid to keep the flies and gnats off, the creature would not allow her to do so. "Finally, I tried doing small circles on his back and side, well away from his head and ear," she explains. She did this twice every day, talking softly to Miso as she drew her circles. Within a few days he became more comfortable with the process.

After two weeks, when she traced larger circles all over his back and shoulders, she was also able to get closer to Miso's ear. "With time, I was able to do small circles on his ears and around the base of the sarcoid, and to remove some of the crust on his face. He would, by then, come to me, stand right next to me, and want the TTouch!" Eventually, her veterinarian came to the house and tied off the sarcoid. After its blood supply had been cut off, the tumor fell off within a few days. Although Miso now has a new sarcoid on his back leg, the one on his ear has not returned.[19]

As with many alternative therapies, there is little but anecdotal evidence that TTouch therapy works, but it has apparently eased pain for many animals, strengthened the human-animal bond, and calmed anxious animals. The practice is currently used by animal guardians, trainers, breeders, veterinarians, and zoo personnel in many countries. Tellington-Jones's Web page (www.lindatellingtonjones.com) includes a directory of practitioners.

REIKI

One complementary technique used quite frequently is Reiki, an ancient Japanese energy healing method that involves the laying on of hands. Reiki, meaning "universal life," has been practiced primarily in Japan and Hawaii, but also in the United States and elsewhere since about 1940. It is a technique particularly effective for producing inner calm and well-being. Some health care facilities now offer Reiki as part of their continuing education curriculum.

Most practitioners believe Reiki was rediscovered in modern times by Mikau Usui, a scholar and mystic from Japan. Usui discovered the formula in obscure Sanskrit writing. After meditating on Mount Kuryama near Kyoto, Japan, for twenty days, Usui received an understanding of the healing properties of this energy renewal system, which he called Reiki.[20] According to Raphaela Pope, an animal Reiki practitioner in Davis, California, the Sanskrit characters received by Usui are sacred and are placed in the aura of all Reiki healers. In addition, Pope says that while Dr. Usui rediscovered, at the end of the nineteenth century, something much older and probably of Tibetan origin, the modern Usui school of Reiki healing started in Japan.[21]

Reiki may be perceived by the client in several ways: as heat, chill, tingling or pulsing sensations, or vibrations, all of which are generally pleasant sensations. Raphaela Pope asserts that "one animal told me that the Reiki treatment was 'like a warm blanket.'" She has found that Reiki for animals with cancer does ease suffering. But she believes animals often find distance healing more useful than hands-on healing. "One can use the distance symbols to send Reiki healing to animals or people far away. . . . I think that many animals find the hands on experience too strong. Often the hands of the Reiki practitioner heat up, and maybe animals find that unpleasant. . . . Reiki is simply sending universal life energy and letting the patient receive and accept it as he or she will."[22]

As Jennah Dickinson, a certified Reiki Master in Texas, explains, "With Reiki, you are helping to attune the energy of a person [or animal]; in contrast, with techniques like massage you are massaging the muscles. . . . You need to have confidence and trust in yourself in order for your connection to happen with animals or humans. Animals know things on a different level than we do. My animals know if I am not into what I am doing and will react accordingly. . . . They live in a whole other world than us."[23]

As she explains in her article "Touch Your Dog," she believes that touching your animals in a meaningful, calm way "builds a sense of safety and confidence" as well as giving them private time with you. She recommends creating a relaxing atmosphere with music that is soothing but not loud. She likes using candles, preferring relaxation aromatherapy candles with a "soft" scent; vanilla works well. A mat or a folded blanket that is comfortable for the dog is a good idea. Initial sessions last five to ten minutes, but this can be increased to thirty minutes daily, depending on the dog. Dickinson starts on the head and neck region, because this is a good place to build trust with the dog. During the massage, she feels for any lumps or abnormalities, so the technique is effective with both well animals and ill ones. Motions are repetitious and gentle.[24]

Dickinson used Reiki on her male rottweiler, Bruhen, after he was diagnosed with pancreatic cancer and given no chance to live. "They wanted to put him on conventional drugs, and I decided to try herbs, Reiki, and acupuncture first before I tried the drugs. We did Reiki three times a day, acupuncture once a day, and herbs every day with his meals." Four years later he died peacefully in his sleep.

Another of Dickinson's dogs, Errybella, a cocker spaniel, was born with a hole in her heart. Her vet gave her no more than a year. The pup turned seven last December. "The vet said that it was a fluke that she lived. I am firmly convinced that it is the Reiki," says Dickinson.

The strongest point in the technique's favor is that it is "excellent for relieving stress, pain, and distress in both the animal and in the person doing the treatment," she explains. Although Dickinson performs Reiki on her own animals—mostly dogs, a few horses, a cow, and one pig (the one cat didn't like it!)—she also does it for a few friends. She adds, though, that "in the small town that I live in Reiki is sort of akin to voodoo." She, however, knows better.

Another Reiki practitioner uses the techniques in her holistic healing practice for animal companions. Betsy Adams has treated more than one hundred clients since 1994. Before she began her work with Reiki, flower essences, kinesiology, color therapy, and homeopathy with animals, she spent fifteen years in biophysics research. Several veterinarians in her area and elsewhere use her services. She has always felt a strong connection to animals: "Animals are my friends. They've been my teachers for years. I watch what they say, what they do. They talk to me."[25]

MASSAGE

The Touch Research Institute of Miami, Florida, has some interesting news about the effect of massage therapy on the immune system. A study was done on HIV-positive men. After about forty-five minutes of massage therapy, five days a week for a month, the men's anxiety and stress decreased. In addition, their numbers of natural killer cells (the first defense of the immune system) increased, suggesting decreased risk for infections such as pneumonia. Might massage have a similar effect for cancer patients? Massage therapy is also known to induce the release of a serotonin-like substance, which might offset the need for chemical-based pain relievers.[26]

At the very least, touch creates bonding and communicates emotion. According to James Burke, a member of the institute's board of directors, "I think we are going to prove that touch helps alleviate disease in animals and humans. Unfortunately, there are a lot of people in our society, children for example, who are deprived emotionally as well as physically, and there are whole sets of diseases that come from that deprivation."[27] I believe Burke's words apply as well to cats and dogs and other animal companions. If deprivation of touch can lead to or exacerbate disease, then certainly it can also, in some way, heal.

16 Pet Insurance and PPOs

One of the reasons that many people do not try a variety of treatment options when their animal companions are stricken with cancer is the expense. The cost of multiple surgeries, radiation, or chemotherapy is often immense, running into thousands of dollars. Then, of course, an animal may need special diets or medications. If you live in a rural area, as I do, you may have to travel frequently to a major city to find a veterinary hospital where your animal companion can receive weekly or monthly radiation or other specialized, state-of-the-art treatments.

This expense is one of the documented reasons that many people don't aggressively treat their animal companions' cancers. Furthermore, according to statistics, veterinary costs in the United States are rising at almost three times the rate of human health care increases: 8.1 percent versus 2.8 percent for humans.[1]

You can easily spend almost as much treating your animal companion's cancer as you can a human disease. Whether to do so comes down to two issues: your ability to pay and your commitment to the animal in question. No one can answer these questions satisfactorily except you. But something has occurred in the past several years to help make these moral and financial dilemmas more palatable and easily solvable for some animal guardians.

It is pet insurance. The concept is wildly popular in countries such as Sweden and England—countries where national health insurance exists, enabling people to spend their income on insuring their animal companions.

In the United States, where approximately forty-five million citizens have no health insurance and many employers are cutting back on insurance coverage, pet insurance has been slower to catch on. But it is catching on—and is certainly not a bad idea if your animal is at risk for cancer.[2] Pet insurance is not a perfect system, but in many cases it may help keep your animal alive and comfortable for a few extra months or years.

VETERINARY PET INSURANCE

Pet insurance became available in the United States in 1982, when Veterinary Pet Insurance (VPI) of California began selling policies. Then-active veterinarian Jack Stephens began the company in 1980. Since that time more than thirty pet insurers have come and gone. VPI remains the largest licensed pet health and accident insurer in the country. VPI covers only dogs and cats. It has sold more than 850,000 policies and enjoys an 82 percent renewal rate. It is licensed in forty-nine states and the District of Columbia.

VPI operates similar to a traditional human health insurer rather than an HMO. Policyholders may choose their veterinarian. The company insures animals eight weeks of age and older; there are no age caps or breed restrictions. After you submit a claim, the average turnaround time is quite short, often about one week. The insurance plan covers such conditions as cancer in dogs, and leukemia and other cancers in cats, if they are not preexisting or "rare congenital or hereditary" types. Aside from surgeries, the policy pays for office calls, prescriptions, treatments, lab fees, X-rays, and hospitalizations for medical problems covered in the individual policy. Alternative treatments such as acupuncture and chiropractic are covered if performed by a licensed veterinarian. Rates are based on the age of the pet and the plan, not on the specific breed.

You can add vaccination and routine care coverage, which pays for annual physical exams, various tests, vaccinations, prescription flea control, dental care, and more. Additional cancer coverage can double your plan's benefit allowances for both canine and feline plans. VPI also offers multiple pet discounts of 5 percent for two to three pets, and 10 percent for four or more enrolled pets. Policies go into effect fourteen days after receipt and acceptance of your application and payment.

According to Dr. Jack Stephens, president of the company, who spoke with me for the first edition of this book in 1999, "Tumors, including cancer, represent over 9 percent of all claims, which is quite high when you consider how many disease categories we have. As a whole group, benign and malignant tumors are second in a group class to skin conditions, such as atopy, pyoderma, etc. Many times a tumor or cancer may be involved [but] not reported to us as such. . . . For example, amputation of the leg could be due to cancer, trauma, or deformity, but we don't always have it reported to us as cancer."[3]

But there's a big catch: Preexisting conditions are not covered by VPI or most pet insurers. If you intend to cover your pets, consider it when they are infants and before they get sick. And, if you purchase insurance from a company other than VPI, read the policy carefully— some cover only accidents for older pets, not illness.

Here are a couple of success stories of people and their pets when insurance helped immensely. Jon Snyder's Great Dane, Jenna, had bone cancer. His veterinarian recommended a procedure "where surgeons remove the cancerous bone and replace it with a donor bone." Snyder carried the Advantage Plus Plan with a cancer endorsement; the procedure cost $10,000 and VPI paid $8,000 of that amount. Snyder might not have proceeded without the policy.[4]

Another satisfied customer is Terry Vinocur, who bought a cancer endorsement because she knew her dog, a boxer named Brooke, is one of several breeds prone to developing cancer. For four years her dog suffered several skin cancers and mast cell tumors. At one point she discovered a tumor "the size of an egg in [Brooke's] thyroid." A specialist removed all the discernible cancer. The surgery and the medications cost $1,200; VPI paid $800 of the claim. "For me, the pet insurance was a godsend," says Vinocur, a policyholder since 1995.[5]

Says Kathy Baumgardner, "Some veterinarians don't support the concept of pet insurance because of the restrictions and exclusions which limit the care a patient can receive while others say pet insurance is the answer to economic euthanasia."[6] Dr. Bruce W. Little, assistant executive vice president of the American Veterinary Medical Association, believes that one reason more Americans are not signing up for veterinary health insurance is their perception that animal care could never push the animal guardian to the brink of bankruptcy the way a human emergency could. Also, adds Dr. Linda Ross, hospital director at Tufts University School of Veterinary Medicine, the lack of coverage for preventive care and preexisting conditions discourages people from buying it.[7]

A NEW OPTION IN THE UNITED STATES

A pet insurance company headquartered in the United Kingdom, and in existence since 1996, offers inexpensive rates and good policies. One of the primary benefits of Healthy Pets Insurance is that it covers not only conventional medicine but also herbal and homeopathic treatments and essential home visits. The company's coverage, available to dogs and cats older than eight weeks, is not breed specific. Animal guardians can use their own vet, and the company will pay 100 percent of claims higher than $80. The policies will not cover preexisting conditions. According to Mark Effenberg, its chief executive, "We are expecting to be promoting a pet insurance programme in the U.S. within the second quarter of this year."[8] The company is underwritten through Lloyds of London, and its staff can give you a quote and let you know when they will be able to cover your animals if you live in the United States.[9] For more information, visit Healthy Pets Insurance's Web site at www.healthy-pets.co.uk.

OTHER COUNTRIES

Kathy Baumgardner also writes of the history of Sweden's pet insurance industry, the oldest and most successful in the world. According to her research, there are about seven hundred thousand dogs in Sweden, 90 percent of whom are purebreds. Of that 90 percent, more than 50 percent are insured by one of seven insurance companies. The company Agria Djurforsakring holds about 70 percent of the pet insurance market and has offered policies for fifty years. It currently insures approximately eighty-five thousand horses and offers plans for cats and parrots, too. This company also offers life insurance policies for pets and loss-of-use policies for working dogs that can no longer perform their work or reproduce. Like VPI, the company covers 80 percent of the claim.

Baumgardner also notes a growth spurt in the pet insurance industry in England. Policies were first offered there in the early 1970s; pet insurance companies design their coverage and set their premiums statistically.[10] Along with Healthy Pets Insurance, described above, British pet insurers include DBI Insurance Company, established in 1947. This company offers two plans for cats and dogs, and another coverage for horses and ponies. If you insure any three dogs and cats (in any combination), you receive a 10 percent discount. The Pet Cover policy for dogs and cats covers items such as accidental death, boarding kennel or cattery fees, a legal helpline for advice on "problems arising from your dog or cat or other matters," "home visits where essential," and the use of herbal and homeopathic remedies. The company's slightly more expensive Premier Cover policy covers loss from illness, disease, or accident; loss by stealing or straying; a legal helpline; home visits and herbal and homeopathic medicines; and more. However, as in the United States, preexisting conditions are not covered.[11]

PPOs

One solution to the lack of coverage for preexisting conditions may be investing in a pet PPO (Preferred Provider Organization). At least this one company in the United States does cover preexisting conditions (including cancer) in a different way than does insurance: Pet Assure, based in Lakewood, New Jersey. The company was begun in late 1996 by Jay Bloom, a former financial officer with Chase Manhattan Bank, who discovered just how expensive animal health care is when his golden retriever, Lucky, needed medical attention. His dog's "inherited condition," hip dysplasia (not uncommon in larger dogs), was not covered by his pet insurance; his bill was $3,000.

Charles Nebenzahl is now president and CEO of the company. Pet Assure's PPO covers any animal of any age—dogs, cats, even a monkey is enrolled. There are no exclusions for preexisting, hereditary, or age-related diseases. There are no waiting periods and no deductibles. They also cover holistic care; even dental care is included. In addition, they will cover any dog, unlike some U.S. pet insurance companies who now refuse to cover what they term "aggressive" dogs.[12]

Here's how the program works. Coverage pays 25 percent of veterinary costs, including surgeries, holistic and alternative care, vaccinations, lab fees, and many other products and services. The 25 percent discount cannot be combined with other discounts. Generally noncovered items include pet food, nonmedical boarding and grooming, and flea products. The program also offers 10 to 50 percent discounts from thousands of participating merchants for some foods, supplies, and grooming services.

To sign up, you pay a $99 annual membership fee for the first animal and $79 for each additional pet. Occasionally, the company runs specials at lower rates. As of late 2004, Pet Assure had close to 2000 veterinarians in 7600 practices in 46 states. Unfortunately the three practices in Vermont are too far from my home for me to be able to make any emergency visits.[13]

As of October 2004, Pet Assure had 100,000 customers and was growing. As stated earlier, the concept has taken a while to be accepted in the United States. "Pet insurance did not start catching on until recently," states Nebenzahl. "The last three years have seen 50% annual growth, but it's still only about 1% of the market."[14] If you have more than one animal, it probably is worth investigating.

INSURANCE FOR ADOPTED ANIMALS

In an announcement on Brakke Consulting, Inc.'s newsletter of December 17, 2004, I found this wonderful, heartwarming news. Here's a more reasonable way to buy your new animal companion insurance, if you adopt him at a shelter. "Pethealth Inc. announced that it has enrolled more than 400,000 dogs and cats in its ShelterCare Pet Insurance Program, and is averaging 23,000 enrollments per month. The program provides a scaled-down insurance package for dogs and cats adopted through Petfinder.com members, with the first 30 days paid for by Petfinder." The ShelterCare Pet Insurance Program is available in Canada and in most U.S. states.[15] The coverage starts at less than $10/month. See www.sheltercare.com/us for more information. Petfinder is one of the largest sites on the Internet where one can find animals available for adoption from shelters around the country. On December 20, 2004, it offered more than 160,000 animals in varying species, sizes, and ages. Included are brief descriptions and a photo.

A DIFFERENT PERSPECTIVE

Not all animal specialists believe that the decision to provide care or not is always based on money. One of my most forthcoming and generous veterinarian experts, Myrna Milani, D.V.M., doesn't hold insurance for her animals, but this is at least in part because she gets all vet services at cost at the clinic where she works. She had this to say about pet insurance: "My big problem with insurers is philosophical," she began. "Its existence is based on a belief in 'financial euthanasia,' i.e., that many people will not consent to treat critically ill and injured animals because they can't afford it." However, she believes this is a myth, based on interviews of many clients for her textbook, *The Art of Veterinary Practice: A Guide to Client Communication* (University of PA Press, 1995). In most cases guardians know the animal best and the decision may be based on not wanting to subject the animal to unnecessary stress. Sometimes they prefer that the animal die at home, in familiar circumstances. When she talks to groups of veterinarians and veterinary students about the human-animal bond, says Milani, "I always tell them to think of it in terms of limits which we all have. For convenience, I mention four groups—time, financial, physical, and emotional/mental. If the veterinarian doesn't address all four of these and the client lacks the confidence to bring them up him/herself, then the chances of owner compliance plummet. If owners recognize that they can't do what the vet wants because of their other limits, they will often say they can't for financial reasons because they believe that's the only one the veterinarian will recognize as real (which maybe is true if his/her education hasn't discussed addressing these other limits, which it often doesn't) or accept as legitimate." She does feel that if the client and the doctor discuss all the limits up-front and all available options, they will be more likely to come up with an appropriate and kind treatment program.[16]

17 If Your Pet Already Has Cancer

Many people will continue to offer their animal companions traditional treatments for cancer—especially surgeries—based on the belief that this will lengthen the animals' lives. If you choose to do so, there are many alternative or strengthening actions you can take after the fact to further extend their time.

Richard Pitcairn, D.V.M., considers several actions critical when your animal companion has cancer. Avoid all commercial foods; feed fresh, unprocessed foods, including a lot of raw foods and organic meat, if available and affordable. Give a lot of vitamin C, half in the morning and half at night. Give oat tincture. Do not give tap water; use filtered, spring-, or distilled water. If a dog or cat becomes ill from radiation or chemotherapy, give cooked oatmeal if possible along with the homeopathic remedy Nux Vomica 6C. And finally, avoid vaccinating your pet.[1]

HILL'S PRESCRIPTION DIET CANINE N/D

One commercial food may be helpful. Available since September 1998, Hill's Prescription Diet canine n/d is formulated specifically for dogs undergoing cancer treatments. (The company earlier developed Hill's Prescription Diet s/d, which helps dissolve bladder stones and crystals in cats, eliminating the need for surgery in many.) Canine n/d is now available nearly worldwide. It is available through many veterinarians, or through the veterinary section of PETsMART stores, but it is not sold on the Internet. The company also offers a toll-free number for questions about their products: (800) 445-5777. Their Web site (www.hillspet.com) contains details of their ongoing research.

Canine n/d contains high levels of n-3 fatty acids, which slow tumor growth; high levels of arginine, which improves immune function; and a patented nutrient profile, which reverses metabolic abnormalities. According to studies published by the scientists who formulated this food, the median survival time for dogs with lymphoma, for example, is 30 days with no treatment; 230 days with chemotherapy and conventional (commercial) food; and 354 days with chemotherapy and canine n/d. The diet is also advertised as able to reverse cancer cachexia (wasting away and malnutrition), reduce side effects of radiation treatments, and prolong remissions. In clinical trials with 273 canine cancer patients, 95 percent of the dogs "readily" ate the product.

But, explains Gregory Ogilvie, D.V.M., professor at Colorado State University, "As with any owner-assisted therapy, the willingness of the pet owner to follow through with treatment is the key to success. This is especially true for cancer patients, because chemotherapy is frequently accompanied by anorexia, nausea, and food aversion." He adds that malnourished dogs do not tolerate surgery or other conventional cancer therapies as well as those on homemade diets.

Canine n/d's ingredients include meat by-products, water, liver, rice, chicken, dried beet pulp, menhaden oil, and various minerals and vitamins. Vitamin E and B_{12} supplements are included. The food should be refrigerated after opening and discarded if not used within thirty-six hours.[2] As of December 2004 its price was approximately $50.49 per 24 cans.

Hill's, which also produces Science Diet (available in specialty pet stores) and Hill's Prescription Diet (available by prescription through veterinarians), has a long history. It was begun in 1948 by veterinarian Mark Morris. Since 1976 it has been a subsidiary of Colgate-Palmolive. The company's products are all extensively tested by veterinarians and scientists. Its Science and Technology Center in Topeka, Kansas, is home to veterinarians, technicians, food scientists, nutritionists, animal care specialists, and others, working in five areas: advanced clinical nutrition, development and commercialization of new products, product improvement, manufacturing and process technology, and professional education.

According to a study by Glenna Mauldin, D.V.M., of Louisiana State University, animals with cancer undergoing radiation treatments who were fed a high-protein, high-fat diet maintained their body weight better than those fed a more typical diet. "Humans undergoing cancer treatment might benefit from the findings in our study, which shows that a highly digestible and energy-dense diet can be effective in maintaining nutritional status," she says.[3]

A large percentage of conventional veterinarians sell the Hill's products, at least in the United States. However, not all practitioners are happy with the company's apparently somewhat aggressive sales tactics. According to an article in *Financial World*, "Hills courts these 'gatekeepers' [veterinarians] the way Neutrogena courted dermatologists to launch its premium priced glycerine soaps. It helps the doctors reap large profits from selling the pet foods."[4] Ann Martin, author of *Foods Pets Die For*, says that many veterinarians are "brainwashed into thinking they have to recommend these commercial foods," because they are repeatedly exposed to them while attending vet school.[5]

One alternative veterinarian I corresponded with did not wish to sell the company's nutritional line; another veterinarian was impressed with the quality of the new canine n/d but preferred to continue to recommend homemade diets to customers over other Hill's products.

OTHER DIETARY THERAPY ADVICE

Gregory Ogilvie, D.V.M., and Antony S. Moore, M.V.Sc., believe dietary therapy can help reverse or eliminate cancer cachexia. Benefits of dietary treatment include weight gain and increased response to and tolerance of other treatments such as radiation, surgery, and chemotherapy. Although the veterinarians admit that the ideal dietary formulation for dogs and cats is not yet known, these are the components they would recommend: "Relatively low amounts of simple carbohydrates, a modest amount of fats (especially omega-3 fatty acids), and adequate amount of highly bioavailable proteins." Although they are writing for veterinarians, their tips might also help you adjust your pet's diet. They also recommend trying several methods to encourage the animal to eat, including warming the food to just below body temperature; providing a variety of tasty and good-smelling foods; and providing stress-free surroundings in which to eat.[6]

Some dogs have been able to live much longer than predicted with a change in diet after diagnosis. Samantha, nicknamed Sam, was a happy reddish golden retriever who lived with an active couple, Mica DiAngelis and Barry Mansfield, in northwestern Vermont. She was a seasoned hiker and traveler, an only companion animal. Like most goldens, she smiled a lot. Sam had always been extremely healthy except for developing hot spots from time to time. As a younger dog, she always got her routinely advised shots, walked and ran long distances, and enjoyed a diet of Blue Seal commercial pet food.

In March 1999, Sam had her routine checkup and was given a combo rabies/distemper shot in her neck. Four or five days later she had her first seizure. The husband was so alarmed, he gave her mouth-to-mouth resuscitation. They thought she might have epilepsy, so the veterinarian gave them steroids for her. She had two or three more seizures, and then they stopped. Sam took steroids for about a month. But she was more lethargic than she had been and not eating as much as previously.

In January 2000, the threesome took off on the southern route for their annual trip to the Southwest. By North Carolina, Sam wasn't doing well at all. Mica and Barry took the dog to a vet who discovered she was extremely anemic. He performed blood tests, an ultrasound, and X-rays. Although he saw no mass, the dog was not producing enough red blood cells, and the veterinarian told the couple that she had bone marrow cancer (a fairly common type of lymphoma in dogs).

An avid animal lover, DiAngelis had been reading Dr. Martin Goldstein's book, *The Nature of Animal Healing,* which advocates many alternative health treatments for animals. Sam's veterinarian had recommended chemotherapy, as she still wasn't eating. A second vet in Florida concurred and said he would like to do a bone marrow test. Sam was almost starving herself at this point. But the couple didn't want to give her chemo or the bone marrow test, considering them too invasive or traumatic.

Based on advice in Goldstein's book, they began to feed her raw beef liver and beef broth. She began to eat again but was still weak and her feces were runny and ugly. Yet another vet pronounced her in very bad shape, and they considered how they would have to bury her in the desert, far from home. By this time, Mica was cooking potatoes to add to the liver and broth. She told me, "And I began talking to her more and doing more massage. She started to eat a bit more. . . . And she didn't die."

They kept increasing Sam's food, adding green vegetables, mostly broccoli, flaxseed oil, fresh garlic, a dog vitamin, and extra vitamin C and E. They changed to a filtered water system. The cooking was time-consuming but worthwhile although they did switch the raw liver to cooked hamburger. Sam, although old and arthritic and almost blind, received a similar diet, to which they added glucosamine, until she died in November 2002. She never had any more vaccinations since that potentially dangerous one in 1999, which meant she could not be licensed (as she had no rabies shot). Her humans felt it was worth the risk; she was alive, joyous, and quite elderly by any standard. Her fur felt better than it had, her ears were in better condition, her breath was fresher and she had good teeth for a 15-year-old lady. She never had hot spots again. The only other additions they added to her diet were a "natural" dog biscuit of lamb and rice and healthy table scraps. She especially enjoyed salad.

Samantha weighed 54 pounds and was still traveling until the end of her life. She went everywhere with her humans and never stayed in a kennel. She took short walks, and she enjoyed an unchanging routine and the enormous love and respect she was paid by her human companions. She was one lucky—and healthy—dog.[7]

LOVE AND A WARM PLACE

If your animal does have cancer, treat her as normally as possible. Of course, diet is critical, and, as we all know, cats are finicky to begin with. Give them some healthy treats if their usual food no longer is appealing. In my experience, our cats and dog with cancer maintained their strength and playfulness for quite some time following surgeries. Most loved to be snuggled. See chapter 15 to read of a cancer patient's experience with Tellington TTouch. This loving massage helped the guardian and her dog bond during the dog's last months.

Cats, especially those old or ill, like warmth and a "room of their own." Author Anita Frazier recommends creating a "snug retreat" consisting of a cardboard box on its side. Put the kitty box in a warm, quiet place. Put a reflector light (seventy-five-watt bulb) nearby; focus it on the box from two feet away. A soft towel or old sweater can become a comfortable mattress. Keep it clean.[8]

REDEFINING *SUCCESS*

Success can mean many things during cancer treatments. For the animal, continuing to have a high quality of life—even a purpose—is critical. Here is one success story.

Kirby, a golden retriever, was a guide dog for Ed Eames, a dog writer and lecturer who became blind in his forties. After his sixth birthday Kirby developed bone cancer (osteosarcoma), and his veterinarian recommended a limb amputation followed by chemotherapy.[9]

Following the operation and chemo, Eames, his wife, Toni, and her golden retriever guide dog, Ivy, began Kirby's rehabilitation. Ivy was particularly important in this process, because the two dogs still ran and played together, fighting over who could catch a ball. Ivy tackled Kirby to get the ball away from him, and, "Facing this challenge, Kirby became agile, learning to twist and sidestep to avoid Ivy's attempts to steal the ball," writes Eames.

Kirby's strength and confidence returned, but Eames did not see how Kirby could continue to be a guide dog. He thought of finding him a retirement home and received many offers. But "the thought of breaking the bond with this marvelous companion and teammate was heart rending." Ed definitely needed an assistance dog to continue his "independence and quality of life." When he was lecturing at the University of California Davis veterinary school, some students suggested the couple try to rehabilitate Kirby as a three-legged guide dog. Although Ed and Toni at first thought this was unrealistic, they decided to give Kirby a chance.

Of course, Eames had to make concessions to his old partner. Kirby needed a new harness, and Eames had to adapt his walking style to his dog's. "Rather than a smooth and gliding motion, there was a bit of a hop to his movement." But Kirby was up to the challenge, and the two continued to travel the United States as Eames lectured to groups about assistance dogs. "As we worked together," writes Eames, "Kirby became a symbol for humans with disabilities." If the dog could work with some minor accommodations, so could people who want to continue leading full lives.

As is all too common, sixteen months after his first diagnosis Kirby's cancer metastasized to his lungs. He became too weak to walk and was euthanized at home. But at least his last year was a happy, productive one. And Kirby will be remembered: He was posthumously inducted into the California Veterinary Medical Association's Animal Hall of Fame.[10]

Then there is Tegan, an Irish setter who had a leg amputated because of bone cancer in June 1995 but was "alive and still kicking" and working as a Delta therapy dog in 2000. As his guardian, Marilyn Putz of Highland Park, Illinois, told me, "Tegan has continued to do well, and we are grateful for each day." The dog was the poster boy for the University of Wisconsin Veterinary Medical School's Oncology Department, which housed the ACT Program. After chemotherapy there, another spot showed up on his lung. He was put back into an experimental phase of chemo, and the spot disappeared. Although the treatment cost "an arm and a leg," says Putz ("no pun intended"), eventually Tegan was accepted into a grant program, and Putz no longer had to pay for his bimonthly checkups. Side effects from Tegan's therapy included an occasional high fever, which was controlled with Ascriptin.

In an update, I learned that Tegan died in 2003 to adenocarcinoma (totally related to his osteosarcoma). "He seemed to have 'the gene,'" said Putz. "He was 11½ years old, eight years older than he was supposed to be when he died." Not only is Tegan honored in this book; he also still graces the cover of the brochure for the ACT Program; and was memorialized in a book about pet therapy, *Therapy Pets: The Animal-Human Healing Partnership* by Jacqueline J. Crawford and Karen A. Pomerinke.[11] Tegan is well remembered.

The Putzes currently live with three Irish setters, none with cancer. They have lost four other setters to cancer—two to osteosarcoma, one to a nasal tumor, and one to a thyroid tumor (she actually died of a heart condition, but her cancer returned after surgery)—so they are overjoyed that Tegan survived as long as he did. Cancer is a major killer among Irish setters.

The best possible ways to prevent cancer and to maintain an old friend who already has it are these: adequate and appropriate exercise, a nutritious diet, caution about pesticides and other environmental risks, caring and current veterinary care, early detection, and lots of love at home.

18 Pain Management for Animals

In the summer of 2004, I witnessed my beloved sister-in-law, Alice, slowly die of cancer. She was in bed for several months, and in pain much longer. She had three surgeries and was on morphine for months. During the three years she had cancer, Alice almost never felt like her original high-spirited and fun-loving self. She was in constant discomfort or pain, although, thankfully, she did take drugs to lessen or alleviate the bulk of it. But even on the day before she died, when she was almost completely uncommunicative, when the Hospice nurse and I turned her over, she cried out a little because it hurt so much.

After experiencing this terrible wasting away and end of a life, I began to realize that I had not adequately addressed pain management in our animals in my first edition. How could I have shortchanged this important piece? Probably for two reasons: it's so much harder to tell if domestic animals are in pain (and they can't actually tell us they are), and only one of our four animal companions who died of cancer seemed to be in any great discomfort. Not one of them was given pain medicine; surely, no one ever gave them morphine. Ought we to have done more?

THE CHALLENGES OF PAIN DETECTION

Many of us are aware of a few signs of pain or discomfort in our companion animals, but we might not be aware of more subtle signs. For example, I notice limping, hot spots, length of toenails, and overall teeth condition, but sometimes I might overlook a totally new symptom for a few days. These oversights can be dangerous, I've learned.

According to the Companion Animal Pain Management Consortium, made up of veterinarians from colleges of veterinary medicine in Colorado, Illinois, and Tennessee, osteoarthritis is the "number one cause of chronic pain in dogs." They estimate that approximately nine million dogs in this country are affected and that approximately 20 percent of those suffer from chronic pain.

The second most common cause of chronic pain in animals is cancer. "Often patients will require a multimodal approach to pain therapy and may be responsive to a variety of nonpharmacologic analgesic therapies (e.g., acupuncture or massage) as well as a number of analgesic adjunctive medications."[1]

Here is the definition of pain, according to the Veterinary Medical Teaching Hospital at the University of Wisconsin, that is used by many veterinarians: "Pain is an unpleasant sensory and emotional experience associated with actual or potential tissue damage."[2] Note the inclusion of "emotional pain."

Rita Reynolds, to whom I frequently refer in this book, has seen her fill of animal pain. She runs an animal sanctuary, Howling Success, in Virginia. Reynolds always lives with between fifteen and twenty animals (plus a husband and a son) in a variety of breeds—cats, dogs, ducks, chickens, donkeys, goats, and a dairy cow. She has dedicated her life to giving these abandoned, often sick and old animals love and comfort for the rest of their lives.

In her work with animals, she is at the forefront of a burgeoning national animal hospice movement. When she is not making special diets, administering shots, or cuddling a creature, she's writing about her experiences in books and in her quarterly journal, *laJoie*.

Over the ten years that I have known her, Reynolds has witnessed at least twenty animals die of cancer. In the fall of 2004, two dogs had cancer, as did one duck. In August 2004, she wrote me the following: "As for pain—animals hide their pain. I learned this the hard way with my birds and Miso, the donkey. They know, instinctively, that to show pain means showing weakness, which means they become vulnerable to attack by predators. So birds and equines, especially, will not show signs of illness, usually, until it is too late—they are nearly dead anyway. I have noticed pain—terrible pain—in the eyes of my dogs, especially Oliver (a small terrier type of dog). It was at that moment, literally, that I rushed him to the animal hospital and told them he needed to be released [euthanized] right then. The animals will show pain by extending their head and neck forward, sometimes arching their necks back and up, and their visual focus becomes non-specific—they no longer focus on the world around them, but you can see they are drawing inward.

"Sometimes an animal will show pain by becoming quiet and withdrawn, or become snappy and even aggressive. A shift in personality is a clear sign something is very wrong. They definitely suffer from severe pain and need medical help with it."[3]

In a later conversation, she added, "Rescue Remedy [see the section on Bach flower remedies in chapter 12] sure does help, but as the cancer progresses, stronger drugs are definitely needed. I keep Valium here on hand, with my veterinarian's permission—a canine dose for a small dog, both rectal valium (for quick results) and tablet form. I do not hesitate for a moment to turn to regular drug therapy or euthanasia if there is severe pain evident due to cancer."[4]

Sadly, the assessment and techniques of pain management have not always received top priority by the veterinary community. They are not alone in underestimating this aspect of care for nonhuman creatures. In fact, quite unbelievable to me, many people didn't even acknowledge that other animals feel pain until Australian philosopher Peter Singer's seminal book, *Animal Liberation* (1975). Even cold-blooded animals feel pain. A study conducted by the Royal Society in England, a charity scientific organization, in early 2003 found that rainbow trout feel pain. The fish in which experimenters injected bee venom or acetic acid in their lips "demonstrated 'rocking' motion, strikingly similar to the kind of motion seen in stressed higher vertebrates like mammals," scientists stated.[5]

In 1999 Brakke Consulting, an American management consulting firm specializing in animal health and related industries, surveyed 146 veterinarians in the United States and discovered that "fewer than 50 percent of practitioners used pain management during routine elective procedures such as spays and castrations. Not all veterinary schools formally address pain management issues and only a few schools offer courses devoted to pain management. Consequently, most practitioners have not received focused training [in this area],"[6] states Charles Short, D.V.M., professor emeritus of anesthesiology and pain management at Cornell University College of Veterinary Medicine and advisor to the Center for the Management of Animal Pain at the University of Tennessee.

Things are not so different in the U.K. In October 2003, Dr. J. C. Brearley, VetMD, Ph.D., presented a paper "Cancer Pain and Analgesia" at a surgical oncology meeting in Cambridge, England. In that paper she writes, "Until recently, and still in some quarters, the effect of cancer pain on quality of life in animals has not been recognized, and so treatment has not been required. If it has been recognized then the most popular option has often been euthanasia with the words 'It is the kindest thing to do.'"[7]

As a side note, in this same paper, Brearley mentioned "nonsteroidal anti-inflammatory drugs" as one class of drugs to use with pain management and "acupuncture" as one physical technique to apply. These are quite different than what is mentioned in U.S. documents I have seen.

ADVANCES IN PAIN MANAGEMENT

But the situation is finally improving for all animals, both family companions and laboratory animals. In 2001, the American Veterinary Medical Association Animal Welfare Forum was dedicated to the topic of pain management. The forum hoped to teach the attending doctors how better to manage and understand pain in dogs and other small animals. An earlier symposium at Cornell University in 1990 brought together 285 participants from 18 countries, states Dr. Charles Short, cochair of that meeting.[8]

Over the last three or four years, animal researchers have become especially keen on learning how better to assess pain. This may be, in part, in reaction to so much attention being paid to human pain. A few of the parameters that scientists look at during observations for amount of pain in animals are these: activity; appearance; temperament; vocalization; feeding behavior; physiological changes; and incision site (where it is swelling, or if the animal is chewing, etc.).[9] As the animals do not speak our languages, "With more subtle evidence we have to trust our intuition and train ourselves to be keen observers," writes Dr. T. J. Dunn in his article, "Managing Pain in Dogs."[10] Reflects Dr. Brearley in her paper entitled "Cancer Pain and Analgesia," "The inability to communicate in no way negates the possibility that an individual is experiencing pain and is in need of appropriate pain relieving treatment."[11]

In early 2004, the Companion Animal Pain Management Consortium, supported by an unrestricted educational grant from Pfizer Animal Health, produced a comprehensive piece, "The Essential Tools for Pain Management," that comes in a mini toolkit-like box. The toolkit consists of a myriad of information about signs and symptoms, about effective drugs (such as codeine, fentanyl, and morphine), about surgical protocols, about veterinary staff strategies, and much more. Members of the consortium included veterinarians from Colorado State University, University of Tennessee, and the University of Illinois at Urbana, and a technical services veterinarian at Pfizer Animal Health, all acknowledged experts in animal pain management.[12]

According to J. Michael McFarland, D.V.M., of Pfizer Animal Health, U.S. Veterinary Operations, this is the first such toolkit produced. An unrestricted educational grant "means that Pfizer provided financial support for the effort, but has no legal control over how the funds are used. . . . the funds were to be used to develop educational tools for veterinary professionals . . . but their ability to use those funds as they see fit in accomplishing that goal is unrestricted." To obtain a copy for their office, veterinarians need to contact Pfizer directly.[13]

There is information in the toolkit that directly relates to pain management for cancer patients. For example, researchers found that cancer pain lies in the moderate to severe pain category and that mass removal of cancerous tissue puts an animal in moderate pain. Bone cancer is in the highest, or "severe to excruciating" pain category. The consortium veterinarians want "clinicians to be more proactive in the assessment of pain . . . and believe that staff members . . . should be an integral part of a pain management team."[14] They agree that "Pain management is individualized for each patient and pain management accompanies all surgical procedures." Drugs such as codeine, fentanyl, and morphine are listed with indication, dose, action, and comments. On the document's second page the operating system of the Consortium is clearly stated: "It is our belief that pain should be considered and evaluated in the same way that we assess a patient's traditional vital signs."[15]

One veterinarian who has long studied pain management in animals, and is part of the consortium, is William Tranquilli, D.V.M., professor of clinical medicine at the University of Illinois, College of Veterinary Medicine, and director of the school's Veterinary Interdisciplinary Pain Service (VIPS), a group of approximately nine doctors in various veterinary specialties, including oncology. He believes that a veterinarian must work hand in hand with the animal's guardian to establish pain management strategies. The veterinarian needs to educate the guardian about his or her animal's needs. "At some point, we have to switch over to quality of life issues, especially if there is no cure. We need to make the remaining life as quality as possible. The veterinarian needs to get as accurate a reading of the pain as possible."[16]

This is especially important with chronic pain, he continues. "Chronic pain in other animals is like chronic pain in humans. Pets will show the people closest to them their pain. The veterinarian needs to better understand the pain and to be able to communicate the level of that pain more clearly to their clients. . . . A veterinarian's role is as an advocate for their patients. People often are psychologically dependent on their pet, especially with an older person who lives alone with one animal. The veterinarian needs to try to break through that kind of relationship and recommend pain management. It's not right to let an animal suffer."

Dr. Tranquilli believes that the veterinary community is dealing with the issue of pain management much more comprehensively than it has in the past, but it still has a ways to go. "I'm hoping, in the long run, the veterinarian community can get this right. We're making inroads with lab animals—we've made huge steps there, but maybe we can become better in treating personal pets in this regard."[17]

Another extremely useful—and necessary—resource to be produced in the last few years is "Management of Animal Pain, Course Syllabus on the Basic Concepts and Clinical Applications." Now in its third edition, it was edited by Charles Short, D.V.M., and is the only such document in existence. The syllabus was prepared by a task force including both U.S. and Canadian colleges, and was funded by Pfizer

Animal Health through a developmental gift sponsored by the consortium mentioned earlier.

Writes Dr. Short, "The management of animal pain is an emerging discipline providing many opportunities for the veterinarian to practice good medicine in either the clinical or research environment. In the past, instruction in pain management for the veterinary student has been segmented within a number of courses within the veterinary college curriculum. Pain is of concern to all veterinarians responsible for animal care. The development and approval of new medications, improved monitoring and measuring technologies, and the use of situation specific protocols for both acute and chronic pain now contribute to our success."[18]

In our correspondence in fall 2004, Dr. Short told me that all veterinary colleges in the United States and Canada have copies of this syllabus, and he believes all the colleges are using it to "some format and extent." He has lectured on pain management in more than thirty countries and received a welcome response. "The movement since 1990 is encouraging and during the last four years, remarkable. We are even making headway in many other countries."[19]

19 Grieving and Accepting the Loss

Losing an animal to cancer is especially difficult. The animal is often in pain, moves awkwardly, and may have large, often visible (sometimes multiple) growths that keep recurring. She may stop eating or no longer want to play. The light may have disappeared from her eyes. You may feel somehow responsible—I did at times—as though you are not giving the proper food, the right water, enough exercise, or whatever you worry about the most. Also, cancer is a huge taboo, a scary word in most people's vocabulary. As Carolyn Ashton, B.V.Sc., wrote me, "There is a lot of shock and fear associated with this [diagnosis]. I hear from people that they didn't hear a word that was spoken by their vet after they said the 'c-word.'"

So grieving an animal's death from cancer can be wrenching. Of course, crying is good for you, and so is having some sort of ceremony to remember the animal when she was younger, healthier, happier. For example, we bury our pets' ashes in our backyard. In our dog Bauhaus's case, we invited our entire cul-de-sac neighborhood to come to this memorial. They shared memories of Bauhaus's life and quirks, and we served popcorn and bananas, her favorite treats. (While buttered popcorn certainly is not good for a dog, bananas, or any fruits, are not bad.)

SOCIAL WORK AND
SUPPORT NETWORKS

The University of Pennsylvania's Veterinary Hospital has a social worker to help animal guardians with the pending loss of an animal to cancer. Just as with human members of the family, when an animal is deathly sick you might have trouble sleeping, or experience memories of previously ill family members or lost loved animal companions. The hospital staff recommends discussing the following with a social worker: hospital procedures; any emotional reaction you may be having; informing other family members, especially small children; decisions about euthanasia; decisions about treatments; your other animals' reactions and how to deal with them; personal problems that may have fallen into the background, such as housing, finances, or school; and translating medical terms so you can understand what is going on.

This hospital also runs a support group that meets every other week for people whose animal companions are ill or have died.[1] I can attest to the power of support groups. Jason is a colleague at the Vermont community college where I teach. When I began writing this book, his dog and cat were both diagnosed with lymphoma. We discussed the prognosis, the treatments, the sorrows. Jason lost both animals—Panda the cat at ten, and Shep the dog at seven—within six months. My husband and I had lost our four animals in the preceding five years. Talking with Jason was immensely helpful; neither of us felt quite so alone.

Anticipating the loss is part of the grieving or letting-go process. A brochure from the University of Illinois College of Veterinary Medicine calls this anticipatory grief. "You may experience anticipatory grief *before* the loss of your companion animal when you learn that your pet has a terminal illness or you weigh the decision to euthanize," it states. The decision to euthanize is especially difficult, both morally and emotionally. Some people choose to hold a party or ritual that might be meaningful to the dying animal.

A recent example comes to mind. You may remember Norton, a Scottish Fold cat who was given to writer Peter Gethers in 1983 and inspired two whimsical books, *The Cat Who Went to Paris* and *A Cat Abroad*. On May 16, 1999, the sixteen-year-old feline died of cancer and kidney failure. Just before Norton's death, Gethers took him to an inn they both enjoyed. "He sat in his chair," says Gethers, "and had a little grapefruit sorbet."[2]

Kansas State University's small-animal clinic has just completed a consultation room furnished like a room in a home. "It's not going to be just a grief room, but a quiet, comfortable and personable room where we can have discussions with clients in a more private atmosphere," says Laura Garrett, veterinarian and assistant professor of oncology. This room is targeted for people whose animal companions have terminal illnesses such as cancer and who need a quiet, contemplative place. "These types of rooms might be good for the animals' well-being as well," Garrett continues. "The pets won't feel like they're still being treated and will maybe relax some because it feels less like a hospital."[3]

ANTICIPATING THE LOSS

Natural therapy veterinarian Carolyn J. Ashton has told me this: "I think that preparation for losing an animal is also part of the healing process and so I include practices such as meditation and animal communication as part of my approach to cancer treatment." She elaborates: "I encourage people to ask their pets to give them a clear sign as to how they want to die (natural or assisted) and when (e.g., is it today?); to give their pet some options so that they can recognize the signs (e.g., I'll know you are ready if you either stop eating or don't wag your tail or look up at us when the family enters the room)." She also uses some natural remedies to aid in this process: "Many ranges of flower essences have one or two that are appropriate for this—for helping communication with nature and spirits, to aid the transition from life through death, and to help one move through the pain of grief."[4]

Donna Raditic, D.V.M., believes that sometimes animal guardians need to let their animal know that it is all right to die. She feels that cats or dogs may stay alive if they know the guardian wants this. "The animal's priorities are most often the more correct ones. The people aren't ready to let go. I can tell if the animal's ready because there's a life force that shines through their eyes. Their eyes have no fear. The owners need to let go; the animals need to hear it's okay to go." She also feels we can learn much from animals about dying, because they are not afraid of death like many of us are. "When animals die, you don't lose something," she reflects. "They are a gift. They're in your heart forever. I may take their body away, but not the gift. They give each one of us something we needed at that time."[5]

Five years later, she reiterated the same message, albeit a bit more emphatically: "Owners experience an incredible lesson about the meaning of life and death. As I often say, 'Animals will teach you how to live and they will teach you how to die'. . . . They want to pass on their simple perspectives on life and let us know that dying is just part of it all."[6]

Reiki Master and animal communicator, Susan Hamlin, of Saratoga Springs, New York, often works with veterinarians during an animal's treatment and, again, when and if it is time for the animal to leave this world. She says "If an animal's journey is to go, communication can help make that an easier path all around, easing fears en route and, if the person wants, communicating with the animal in spirit afterwards to reassure the person that all is well. Animals tend to be much easier passing over and back than humans," she continues. "Even with their fierce survival instinct, they seem to accept that death is a part of the whole picture and get on with it. My dear old black lab Luther (who had mast cell cancer but lived with it, with the help of an integrative approach, for six years with no surgery) paid a quick but exuberant 'visit' to me at the Irish Pub where we hoisted pints in his honor an hour after his last trip to the vet. Talk about confirmation that all is well in this life and beyond!"[7]

OTHER ANIMALS MOURN, TOO

Another factor to consider about grieving or mourning a lost animal companion is that the remaining animals in the home often grieve as well. It is quite clear that animals grieve the loss of a human (my mother's cat was depressed for weeks after my father died—lying on Dad's favorite flannel shirt helped somewhat), but they also grieve their animal companions. The ASPCA Companion Animal Mourning Project study in 1995 showed that it is not only people who become depressed or despondent when a loved animal dies.

According to this study, 58 percent of cats and dogs became more affectionate, some even becoming clingy, after the death of another animal in the home. A reported 70 percent of cats and 63 percent of dogs meowed or barked differently; 46 percent of cats and 36 percent of dogs ate less than usual. And, overall, 65 percent of cats and 66 percent of dogs exhibited four or more behavioral changes, which generally lasted from between one and six months. In the study Paula Anreder notes that owners frequently try to share the process with the remaining animals. Some even show the dead body to the animal companions, believing this is helpful.[8]

Television personality George Page writes in his first book about one of his dogs, Mink, a golden retriever. When Mink's mother, Jenny, died (they lived together in the Page household), Mink "looked and sniffed at Jenny's body and clearly did not have the slightest idea what to make of it. When we took Jenny's body outside to the grave we dug behind the house, Mink acted as though she had lost her mind." The younger dog ran around the yard so much she finally "dropped from sheer exhaustion." Following the burial, Mink would not leave her humans alone for a minute. But her loss seemed to hit her fully within two or three days, "when she just stopped eating, lay down, and paid no attention to anyone or anything." This alarming activity continued for about two weeks, until the Pages decided a new companion might help Mink recover. They adopted a yellow Labrador puppy named Maggie. Over the course of Maggie's first day, the two canines bonded and became inseparable until Mink died years later.[9]

In her book *The Heart That Is Loved Never Forgets: Recovering from Loss: When Humans and Animals Lose Their Companions,* author and animal healer Kaetheryn Walker addresses this topic. She notes that many animals' changed behaviors may remind us of our own process of grieving. In her work with animals she often recommends a variety of homeopathic remedies for the grieving animals remaining in the family. These include aconitum, gelsemium, phosphorus, and stramonium for severe panic. Bach Flower Calming Essence (also called Nature's Rescue) can also calm, especially during initial grief. Another remedy Walker recommends for animal use is the herb and flower essence formula Broken Heart Remedy, made by Avena Botanicals (see the resources).[10]

COUNSELING SERVICES

A variety of bereavement counseling services and hotlines exist, at least in the United States, for those who will lose or have lost an animal companion. The ASPCA Counseling Department in New York City, an official Delta Society affiliate, for instance, offers several services. The first is twenty-four-hour free access to a psychologist, Stephanie LaFarge, senior director of counseling services, via her beeper at (800) 946-4646. If you punch in pin number 140-7211 and then your phone number, she will return your call. The ASPCA assumes all phone costs. She also offers face-to-face counseling services in her office at the ASPCA in New York City and runs a group, on an as-needed basis, for children whose pets have died. You may contact the office via the ASPCA's Web site www.aspca.org or by phone at (212) 876-7700 ext. 4355. The Animal Medical Center in New York City also has a counseling program and runs a pet loss support group. For more information call (212) 838-8100.

The University of Illinois College of Veterinary Medicine, offers the C.A.R.E. (Companion Animal Related Emotions) Helpline. Trained veterinary student volunteers answer the phone personally on Tuesday, Thursday, and Sunday between 7 and 9 P.M. Central Time, and calls are returned. There is no charge for the service, although, of course, donations in memory or in honor of a beloved pet are appreciated. The toll-free number is (877) 394-2273. They also have a Web site with further information, including book recommendations, www.cvm.uiuc.edu/CARE.

According to Andrea Lynn Morden-Moore, student director of the C.A.R.E. Helpline, "We offer a compassionate ear to people who have either lost a companion animal, or are anticipating a loss. About a third of our callers are horse owners. The bulk of our calls, however, are from cat and dog owners." She understands such worries and grieving. Her ten-year-old French bulldog, Gnarly, first developed a cancerous rectal polyp at age five. It was surgically resected, or severed, at the base. Then, at eight, he developed a lump on his shoulder, eventually diagnosed as a spindle cell sarcoma. After surgery and daily radiation for a month, Gnarly regained his weight and is now more energetic and happy. "People need to know that cancer isn't necessarily a death sentence. If the cancer cannot be beaten, at least people can have more time to prepare for their losses, and to say good-bye," Morden-Moore reiterates.

Michigan State University offers both a hotline and support group. According to Sally Walshaw, V.M.D., of Pet Loss Support Programs, the program's hot line, in existence since 1994, is open on Tuesday, Wednesday, and Thursday from 6:30 to 9:30 P.M. Eastern Time, staffed by College of Veterinary Medicine student volunteers. Call (517) 432-2696. The Pet Loss Support Group, established in 1992, meets on the first Tuesday of each month at 7 P.M. in Room A-174 of the Small Animal Hospital at the university. A professional counselor assists people in dealing with the loss of a companion animal.

The Pet Grief Support Service of the Companion Animal Association of Arizona (a volunteer-based agency dealing with therapy animals) helps people throughout the United States and Canada who are anticipating or coping with the loss of an animal companion. The group offers a twenty-four-hour-a-day telephone helpline staffed by trained volunteer counselors, support group meetings, literature, and more. You can reach Pet Grief Support Service at (602) 995-5885. They also run an ongoing support group for grieving animal lovers on the first Saturday of every month from 9:00 to 10:30 A.M. in Conference Room 1 at the Hospice of the Valley, 1510 East Flower Street, in Phoenix.[11] For more information visit their Web site at www.caaainc.org/petgriefsupport.htm.

Dr. Ashton tells me that she often uses meditation practices for people "still aggrieved by a past decision regarding a pet."[12] For example, guardians may sit in meditation on the beach, in the woods, or at a table in their homes with aids such as "the pet's ashes, their photos, their blanket or favorite toy." Ashton believes this practice will bring the animal companion back into their awareness: "They then ask their pet for forgiveness, for what they feel may have been a 'wrong' decision, and then when that is received (which it always will be) to ask themselves for the same forgiveness." As she often does, she may recommend certain Bach flower remedies in this type of situation.

Dr. Ashton tries to help her clients maintain some connection with their deceased companion animal and some hope for the future. "For many people, losing a pet means losing what they see as the strongest and most palpable expression of unconditional love that they have experienced. . . . So regardless of the terms and words that you use (angels, spirits, souls, etc.) I think the importance is to remind people what they already know underneath their overwhelming fear: that they will still have access to this unconditional love even without the animal there in physical form, and that the experience can and will come to them again, if they can keep their heart open."[13]

A national group first dedicated solely to dogs with cancer is the National Cancer Society for Animals (NCSA). Andrea Spencer, of Norton, Massachusetts, is its founder and president. She lost her "miracle dog" Professor, a Weimaraner, to cancer and now lives with six of his relatives. Professor was given two months to live but continued on for two years with both conventional and alternative treatments and lots of love. Although originally only for dogs, explains Spencer, "A few months into our support phone-line establishment, a man in Florida called about his horse. He had heard by an Internet connection that someone out there was holding the hands of panicking animal owners. Why would I not offer him comfort? From there it became ferrets, cockatiels, monkeys—anyone who could fit onto the ark had my ticket." The NCSA operates a 24-hour hotline, offers doctors' office companionship visits, outreach, and education, and sponsors related events such as parades and exhibits.[14]

If you want to celebrate and remember your animal companions in a more formal, national way, a "holiday" has been established for just such memories. National Pet Memorial Day is held on the second Sunday of September. Sponsored by the International Association of Pet Cemeteries, its activities include open houses at participating cemeteries, candle-lighting vigils and other remembrance services. Military, police, and fire canines are especially cited, as well. The cemeteries are in the United States, Australia, Canada, England, and the Virgin Islands.[15] (For a list of pet cemetery members, go to www.iaopc.com.)

Finally, a fairly new but growing phenomena is newspapers that run obituaries for animals. One of our Vermont papers, the daily Times Argus, began this kind practice in August 2004. As its managing editor Maria Archangelo explained, "We figured they are part of the family and we should give people the opportunity to talk about that."[16] Seeing an obituary of any loved one and sharing and saving it does provide a certain amount of closure in these lonely times.

READING ON GRIEVING

Several good books exist on grieving your lost companion. Two I can recommend are *Beyond the Rainbow Bridge* by Rita Reynolds and *Preparing for the Loss of Your Pet—Saying Goodbye with Love, Dignity, and Peace of Mind* by Myrna Milani, both of whom I quote extensively in this book.

One of my all-time favorites is *Goodbye, Friend: Healing Wisdom for Anyone Who Has Ever Lost a Pet* by Gary Kowalski. He reinforces the importance of planning a ritual or ceremony when a pet dies: "Our sense of loss needs to be respected, not belittled," he writes, especially if anyone attempts to minimizes the loss.[17] The final section of his book includes poems and readings, ranging from the Bible to Emily Dickinson to the Koran, that can be used at such ceremonies. As Kowalski tells us, "For some people, the death of a pet may represent the greatest loss they have ever encountered."[18]

In total, the book is not only about healing when a cat, dog, or ferret dies. Rather, it reasserts Kowalski's primary message that animals are important, that "pets are not petty,"[19] that they deserve our respect and our kind care.

Conclusion

As I noted in my introduction, I wrote the first edition of this book after we lost four animals, over a short period of time, to various cancers. We had not neglected our animal companions or treated them badly. I wanted to get to the bottom of this. Of course, I found no one solution or answer, because cancer is complex and comes in many varieties. But once I completed my extensive research for this book, some of my previous suspicions, which I will share below, were confirmed.

I am most happy to report that all three of our current animal companions—Wanda, Bruno, and Stella—have so far had no lumps or bumps, and I have greatly benefited from the research I did for the book; so have they. Their lives are probably quite a bit better than were the four who died, although they all were greatly loved. Here's what I still believe, even more than I did five years ago:

+ We humans can do much more to prevent many animal cancers. We can feed our animals a more nutritious and balanced natural diet. We can be more judicious about using vaccines and flea and other commercial health care products. We can take more control over what environmental toxins our animals are exposed to. We can lower the stress level of our pets, in part by lowering our own stress, and we can become better human-animal communicators. We can spend more time with our animals, and we must take them into our homes forever—not just for a short time until they are inconvenient.

+ It is critically important to choose veterinary care based on full knowledge of that person's background, philosophy, and experiences. We should get our pets started on the right paw immediately. We should shop around and, if our animals do get sick, get second or third opinions, just as we now do with our own doctors.

+ To my great joy, many new options exist if an animal is diagnosed with cancer. Today, many alternative or complementary therapies can go hand in hand with the conventional three: surgery, radiation, and chemotherapy. Many veterinarians are using both types of medicine to enable our animal companions to lead longer, more comfortable lives. The number of alternative-minded veterinarians is increasing—and more people are doing whatever it takes to make their animals healthier and happier.

+ Too often cancer means that death is inevitable in the near future—but not always. Even if an animal will live only one year, that year can be rich and tender. And even if death is imminent, we can help ensure that the remainder of our animals' lives are more healthy and productive. They can teach us, along the way, how to deal better with grieving and with dying.

I believe we need to consider redefining the term *success* in the cancer arena. Veterinarians and health care practitioners can occasionally cure cancers, but they more frequently palliate and treat the symptoms. Prevention and early detection, as is true with human cancers, are vital. With lifestyle changes, our animals can live longer lives in less pain. *Success* in cancer may not involve a long-term, permanent cure. The word may mean something different—less pain, more joy, and, if necessary, learning to know when it is time to let go.

Resources

Abady Food, dry and canned dog food and supplements, 201 Smith Street, Poughkeepsie, NY 12601; (914) 473-1900.

Academy of Veterinary Homeopathy, P.O. Box 9280, Wilmington, DE 19809; (866) 652-1590; www.theavh.org.

Acorn Supplements, Ltd., specializes in natural products for animals, specifically cats and dogs. Their products have been developed in close liaison with veterinarians, animal nutritionists, and dieticians. They supply products worldwide. P.O. Box 103, Robertsbridge, East Sussex, TN32 5ZT, United Kingdom; 01580-881333; fax: 01580-881444; www.acorn-supplements.co.uk.

AltVetMed, Web site for all alternative, complementary, and holistic veterinary medicine, www.altvetmed.org.

The American Holistic Veterinary Medical Association, includes a referral directory, which lists practitioners by state and in Canada along with the modalities they practice, 2218 Old Emmorton Road, Bel Air, MD 21015; (410) 569-0795; e-mail: office@ahvma.org; www.ahvma.org.

American Veterinary Chiropractic Association, 442154 E. 140 Road, Bluejacket, OK 74333; (918) 784-2231; e-mail: amvetchiro@aol.com.

Animal Concerns Community, part of EnviroLink Network. A huge Web site dedicated to the welfare and rights of wild and domestic animals, www.AnimalConcerns.org.

Animal Radio Network, weekly show on several stations throughout the country. Also, a newsletter with sound on the Web, www.animalradio.com.

Animals' Apawthecary, run by Mary Wulff-Tilford and Greg Tilford, herbalists and authors of *All You Ever Wanted to Know About Herbs for Pets,* P.O. Box 131388, Carlsbad, CA 92013; www.animalessentials.com; e-mail: info@animal essentials.com.

Ark Naturals, Natural Products for Pets, all-natural, holistic pet care products, Gulf Coast Nutritionals, Inc., 6166 Taylor Road, #105, Naples, FL 34109; (800) 926-5100; fax: (239) 592-9338; www.arknaturals.com.

ASA Pet Supplies, Inc., holistic pet treat supplements, 38 Carnforth Road, North York, Ontario, M4A, 2K7, Canada; (239) 592-9338.

ASPCA Animal Poison Control Center, a consultation fee may apply, 1717 S. Philo Road, Suite 36. Urbana, IL 61802, (888) 426-4435; www.apcc .aspca.org.

Avena Botanicals, organically grown herbal products for dogs and cats, herb gardens, herb courses, 219 Mill Street, Rockland, ME 04856; (207) 594-0694; www.avenaherbs.com.

Lisa Ayala, certified herbalist and iridologist, P.O. Box 26796, San Jose, CA 95159; (408) 244-7200.

B-Naturals, natural and holistic supplements and consultations for dogs and cats, includes products specifically for cancer patients (can ship overseas), P.O. Box 217, Rockford, MN 55373; (866) 368-2728; fax: (763) 477-9588; www.b-naturals.com. For product information and consultations, call Lew Olson at (207) 392-3935.

Cancer Control Society, dedicated to alternative health care options. Annual convention every Labor Day weekend features latest findings in cancer treatment, 2043 N. Berendo St., Los Angeles, CA 90027; (323) 663-7801; fax: (323) 663-7757; www.cancercontrolsociety.com.

D'Arcy Naturals, herbal pet care products and acupuncture, (800) RXDARCY (800) 793-2729.

The Delta Society, a membership society celebrating animal companions and therapy animals. Bookstore, conferences, magazine, 875 124th Avenue N.E., Suite 101, Bellevue, WA 98005; (425) 226-7357; www.deltasociety.org.

Denes Natural Pet Care Limited, pet foods, herbal medicines, and aromatherapy products. Except food, products can be ordered from overseas via the company's Web site. Denes can also provide a list of veterinary surgeons in England using complementary therapies, 2 Osmond Road, Hove, East Sussex BN3 1BR, England; +44 (0) 1273 325364; fax: +44 (0) 1273 325704; www.denes.com.

Dr. Goodpet Pet Pharmacy, Natural Pet Pharmacy for Dogs and Cats, homeopathic medicines, vitamins and minerals, digestive enzymes, flea control products, shampoos, and books, P.O. Box 4547, Inglewood, CA 90309; (800) 222-9932; fax: (310) 672-4287; www.goodpet.com.

EarthRider Laboratories, formulas for pets; a homeopathic kit for animals and people, P.O. Box 3805, Boulder, CO 80307-3805; (303) 543-9888; e-mail: psyched@diac.com.

Green Hope Farm, flower essences featuring an animal wellness collection of twenty-two remedies, free informational guide upon request, Green Hope Farm, POB 125, Meriden, NH 03770; (603) 469-3662; fax: (603) 469-3790; e-mail: green.hope.farm@valley.net; www.greenhopeessences.com.

Halo, Purely for Pets, foods, herbal remedies, vitamins, and more, 3438 East Lake Road, Suite 14, Palm Harbor, FL 34685; (800) 426-4256; www.halopets.com.

Holistic Animal Therapy Association of Australia (HATAA), an association of animal therapists, formed in 1998, who use a variety of holistic healing methods, www.hataa.asn.au.

holisticpet.com, cat and dog health resources and store, www.holisticpet.com.

Hugs for Homeless Animals, a comprehensive Web site that contains a worldwide animal shelter directory, a worldwide list of lost and found pets, a bookstore, a kids connection, and more, www.h4ha.org.

In Defense of Animals, a nonprofit animal advocacy organization, 131 Camino Alto, Mill Valley, CA 94941; (415) 388-9641; fax (415) 388-0388; www.idausa.org.

International Society for Animal Rights, founded in 1959, a leader in the field of animal rights, 965 Griffin Pond Road, Clarks Summit, PA 18411; (800) 543-ISAR; fax: (570) 586-9580; www.isaronline.org.

International Veterinary Acupuncture Society (IVAS), a nonprofit organization related to veterinary acupuncture, P.O. Box 271395, Fort Collins, CO 80527; (970) 266-0666; fax: (970) 266-0777; www.ivas.org.

interPET Laboratories, natural, organic grooming products, 7517 Northwest 41 Street, Coral Springs, FL 33065; (800) 249-2254.

Karma, organic dog food (See Natura Pet Products), www.karmaorganic.com.

Morris Animal Foundation, established in 1948, the largest nongovernmental foundation in the United States that supports studies for dog and cat cancers,

45 Inverness Drive East, Englewood, CO 80112-5480; www.morrisanimal foundation.org.

Natura Pet Products, natural pet products, mainly foods, P.O. Box 271, Santa Clara, CA 95052; (800) 532-7261; www.naturapet.com.

Pet Medicine Chest, natural health products for rabbits, birds, dogs, cats, and horses; www.petmedicinechest.com.

PetPlace.com, a Web site of "news, health and well-being" written and edited by veterinarians. In conjunction with some of the top veterinary colleges and hospitals, www.petplace.com.

Pets 911, a free network recently coupled with The Animal Planet. "Find, adopt, or help a pet where you live." Also lists shelters, clinics, and veterinarians. Toll-free, bilingual, (888) PETS-911; www.pets9ll.com.

PetSage, "a new wisdom in pet care" Web site. Holistic and healthy choices of all sorts—toys, food, books, (800) PET-HLTH (738-4584); www.petsage.com.

Pets with Disabilities, c/o Double Ds, 1010 Theater Drive, Prince Frederick, MD 20678; (410) 257-3141.

Pet Theft Hotline, (800) STOLEN PET.

Springtime, Inc., natural supplements for horses, dogs, and humans, including food concentrates, herbal extracts, and more, 10942-J Beaver Dam Road, P.O. Box 1227, Cockeysville, MD 21030; (800) 521-3212; fax: (410) 771-1530.

The Veterinary Cancer Society, a nonprofit educational organization formed in 1976 by a group of veterinary oncologists, P.O. Box 1763, Spring Valley, CA 91979; www.vetcancersociety.org.

VetQuest, a Web site with basic information on more than twenty-five thousand U.S. veterinary hospitals and clinics, www.vetquest.com.

Victoria's Pet Nutrition Center and Boutique, 25-A N. Main Street, Fond du Lac, WI 54935; (920) 923-1991; www.allnaturalpethealth.com.

Wolfsong Natural Herbal Products, Route 1, Box 357, Wingina, VA 24599; (877) 478-9769; www.wolfsongherbs.com.

The Woof Gazette Dog Magazine, with Uncle Matty, Matthew Margolis. News, features, and pet care information, www.unclematty.com/woofpub.

Wysong Corporation, dog and cat foods, litter, shampoos, and more, 1880 North Eastman Street, Midland, MI 48642; (989) 631-0009; fax: (989) 631-8801; www.wysong.net.

Recommended Reading

Anderson, Nina, and Howard Pieper. *Are You Poisoning Your Pets? A Guidebook to How Our Lifestyles Affect the Health of Our Pets.* Garden Park City, N.Y.: Avery Publishing Group, 1998.

Anderson, Robert, D.V.M., and Barbara Wrede. *Caring for Older Cats and Dogs: Extending Your Pet's Healthy Life.* Charlotte, Vt.: Williamson Publishing, 1990.

Animal Wellness Magazine, "devoted to natural health in animals," 164 Hunter Street W., Peterborough, ON K9H 2L2, Canada; www.animalwellnes magazine.com.

The Bark, a literary and informative quarterly dog magazine, 2810-8th Street, Berkeley, CA 94710; (510) 074-0827; fax: (520) 704-0933; www .thebark.com.

Best Friends Magazine, published by the United States' largest sanctuary for abused and abandoned animals, Best Friends Animal Sanctuary, Kanab, UT 84741-5001; (435) 644-2001; www.bestfriends.org.

Billinghurst, Dr. Ian, B.V.Sc. *Give Your Dog a Bone: The Practical Commonsense Way to Feed Dogs for a Long Healthy Life.* New South Wales, Australia, 1993; and *Grow Your Pups on Bones,* both available at www.herbal-dogkeeping.com.

Birr, Ursula, Gerald Krakauer, and Daniela Osiander. *Dog's Best Friend: Journey to the Roots of an Ancient Partnership.* Rochester, Vt.: Park Street Press, 1999.

Brennan, Mary L., D.V.M., with Norma Eckroate. *The Natural Dog: A Complete Guide for Caring Owners.* New York: Plume Books/Penguin, 1994.

Carson, Rachel, *Silent Spring,* 1962. Reprint, Boston: Houghton Mifflin, 1987.

Catnip, produced by the Tufts School of Veterinary Medicine, a monthly cat newsletter. For subscriptions, contact Customer Service Department, P.O. Box 420014, Palm Coast, FL 32142-0014; www.vec.tufts.edu/vetgeneral/ newsletters/Catnip.html.

Cohen, Carl and Tom Regan. *The Animal Rights Debate.* Walnut Creek, Calif.: Rowman & Littlefield Publishers, Inc., 2001.

Desmond Morris. *Dogs, The Ultimate Dictionary of Over 1,000 Dog Breeds.* North Pomfret, Vt.: Trafalgar Square Publishing, 2001.

Eat, Drink, and Wag Your Tail, DVD about dog nutrition, featuring Dr. Richard Pitcairn. Produced and directed by Pamela Berger. Los Angeles: Interdependent Pictures. www.idpics.com or e-mail idpics@adelphia.net.

Frazier, Anita, with Norma Eckroate. *The New Natural Cat: A Complete Guide for Finicky Owners.* Rev. ed. New York: Dutton/Penguin, 1990.

Glen, Samantha. *Best Friends: The True Story of the World's Most Beloved Animal Sanctuary.* Introduction by Mary Tyler Moore. New York: Kensington Publishing Corporation, 2001.

Goldstein, Martin, D.V.M. *The Nature of Animal Healing: The Path to Your Pet's Health, Happiness, and Longevity.* New York: Alfred A. Knopf, 1999.

Goodall, Jane, and Marc Bekoff. *The Ten Trusts. What We Must Do To Care for the Animals We Love.* HarperSanFrancisco, 2002.

Goodall, Jane, with Phillip Berman. *Reason for Hope.* New York: Warner Books, 1999.

Grim, Randy. *Miracle Dog.* Loveland, Colo.: Alpine Blue Ribbon Books, 2005.

Harriman, Marinell. *House Rabbit Handbook: How to Live with an Urban Rabbit.* Rev. ed. Alameda, Calif.: Drollery Press, 1991.

Hillyer, Elizabeth V., D.V.M., and Katherine E. Quesenberry, D.V.M. *Ferrets, Rabbits and Rodents: Clinical Medicine and Surgery.* Philadelphia: W. B. Saunders, 1997.

Hogan, Linda, Deena Metzger, and Brenda Peterson, eds. *Intimate Nature: The Bond Between Women and Animals.* New York: Fawcett Columbine, 1998.

Howey, Paul M. Freckles. *The Mystery of the Little White Dog in the Desert.* Phoenix: AZTexts Publishing, Inc., 2003.

Knapp, Caroline. *Pack of Two: The Intricate Bond Between People and Dogs.* New York: Bantam Dell Publishing Group, 1998.

Kowalski, Gary. *The Bible According to Noah, Theology as if Animals Mattered.* New York: Lantern Books, 2001.

———. *Goodbye, Friend: Healing Wisdom for Anyone Who Has Ever Lost a Pet.* Walpole, N.H.: Stillpoint Publishing, 1997.

————. *The Souls of Animals.* 2d ed. Walpole, N.H.: Stillpoint Publishing, 1999.

Kübler-Ross, Elisabeth. *On Death and Dying.* New York: MacMillan, 1970.

laJoie, *The Journal That Honors All Beings,* quarterly journal, laJoie and Company, P.O. Box 145, Batesville, VA 22924; (540) 456-6204.

Lane, Marion S., et. al. *Complete Guide to Dog Care, The Humane Society of the United States.* New York: Little, Brown, 1998.

Lazarus, Pat. *Keep Your Dog Healthy the Natural Way.* New York: Fawcett Books, 1999.

Lloyd-Jones, Buster. *Come into My World: Animals and Other People.* London: Martin Secker and Warburg, 1972.

Lufkin, Elise. *Found Dogs: Tales of Strays Who Landed on Their Feet.* Hoboken, N.J.: Howell Book House, 1997.

Mahoney, James, D.V.M. *Saving Molly: A Research Veterinarian's Choices.* Chapel Hill, N.C.: Algonquin Books, 1998.

Martin, Ann. *Food Pets Die For: Shocking Facts about Pet Food.* Troutdale, Oreg.: NewSage Press, 1997.

————. *Protect Your Pet, More Shocking Facts.* Troutdale, Ore.: NewSage Press, 2001.

McGinnis, Terri, D.V.M. *The Well Dog Book: The Classic Comprehensive Handbook of Dog Care.* New York: Random House, 1991.

Milani, Myrna M., D.V.M. *The Art of Veterinary Practice: A Guide to Client Communication.* Philadelphia: University of Pennsylvania Press, 1995.

————. *Preparing for the Loss of Your Pet: Saying Goodbye with Love, Dignity, and Peace of Mind.* Rockland, Calif.: Prima Lifestyles, 1998.

Mills, Linda E., ed. *Current Veterinary Therapy XI: Small Animal Practice.* Philadelphia: W. B. Saunders, 1992.

Mindell, Earl, and Elizabeth Renaghan. *Earl Mindell's Nutrition and Health for Dogs.* Rocklin, Calif.: Prima Publishing, 1998.

Mooney, Samantha. *A Snowflake in My Hand.* New York: Delacorte Press, 1983.

Orey, Cal. *The Essential Guide to Natural Pet Care for Cats and Dogs: Cancer.* Irvine, Calif.: Bowtie Press, a Division of Fancy Publications, 1998.

Page, George. *Inside the Animal Mind.* New York: Doubleday, 1999.

A Passion for Dogs: The Dogs Home Battersea. Forewords by Katie Boyle and Desmond Morris. Introduction by Prince Michael of Kent. Newton Abbot, Devon, England: David and Charles Publishers, 1992.

Pinney, Chris C., D.M.V. *The Illustrated Veterinary Guide for Dogs, Cats, Birds and Exotic Pets.* New York: TAB Books, McGraw-Hill, 1992.

Pitcairn, Richard H., D.V.M., and Susan Hubble Pitcairn. *Dr. Pitcairn's*

Complete Guide to Natural Health for Dogs and Cats. Rev. ed. Emmaus, Penn.: Rodale Press, 1995.

Plechner, Alfred J., D.V.M., with Martin Zucker. *Pets at Risk: From Allergies to Cancer, Remedies for an Unsuspected Epidemic.* Troutdale, Ore.: NewSage Press, 2003.

Puotinen, C. J. *The Encyclopedia of Natural Pet Care.* Lincolnwood, Ill.: Keats Publishing, NTC/Contemporary Publishing, 1998.

———. *Natural Remedies for Dogs and Cats.* Berkeley, Calif.: Publishers' Group West, 1999.

Reynolds, Rita. *Blessing the Bridge: What Animals Teach Us about Death, Dying, and Beyond.* Troutdale, Oreg.: NewSage Press, 2000.

Roth, Melinda. *The Man Who Talks to Dogs: The Story of Randy Grim and His Fight to Save America's Abandoned Dogs.* New York: St. Martin's Griffin, 2004.

Schneck, Marcus, and Jill Caravan. *Cat Facts.* Rockleigh, N.J.: Barnes and Noble Books, 1993.

Schoen, Allen M., D.V.M., M.S. *Kindred Spirits: How the Remarkable Bond Between Humans & Animals Can Change the Way We Live.* New York: Broadway, 2002.

Schultze, Kymythy, R. *Natural Nutrition for Dogs and Cats: The Ultimate Pet Diet.* Carlsbad, Calif.: Hay House, 1999.

Schwartz, Cheryl, D.V.M. *Four Paws Five Directions: A Guide to Chinese Medicine for Cats and Dogs.* Berkeley, Calif.: Celestial Arts, 1996.

Shefferman, Mary R. *An Owner's Guide to a Happy Healthy Pet: The Ferret.* New York: Howell Book House, 1996.

Strombeck, Donald R., D.V.M. *Home-Prepared Dog and Cat Diets: The Healthful Alternative.* Ames: Iowa State University Press, 1999.

Thurston, Mary Elizabeth. *The Lost History of the Canine Race: Our 15,000-Year Love Affair with Dogs.* Kansas City: Andrews and McMeel, 1996.

Tobias, Michael, and Kate Solisti-Mattelon, eds. *Kinship with the Animals.* Hillsboro, Oreg.: Beyond Words Publishing, 1998.

Walker, Kaetheryn. *The Heart That Is Loved Never Forgets.* Rochester, Vt.: Healing Arts Press, 1999.

———. *Homeopathic First Aid for Animals: Tales and Techniques from a Country Practitioner.* Rochester, Vt.: Healing Arts Press, 1998.

The Whole Dog Journal. For subscriptions, write to 75 Holly Hill Lane, Greenwich, CT 06830-6077. For customer service: (800) 424-7887.

Working Dogs Cyberzine, www.workingdogs.com.

Yankee Dog, a quarterly paper for the Northeast. Bowser Publications, P.O. Box 144, Jacksonville, Vermont 05342; (802) 368-7660; www.bowserpublications.com.

APPENDIX C

Glossary

If you do not understand the terminology your veterinarian is using, always ask him or her to explain it in lay terms. As is true when you are discussing human health situations, you must understand the treatments that are proposed in order to be able to make the wisest and kindest decisions for your pet and for your family.

Much of the following glossary comes from OncoLink, an excellent Web site of the University of Pennsylvania Cancer Center. The definitions of *neoplasm, oncology, palliate,* and *partial remission* come from Hill's Pet Nutrition company literature.

Adenoma: A benign epithelial tumor.

Allopathic medicine: "Conventional" medicine in which doctors treat disease through drugs, chemicals, and surgeries rather than focusing on prevention or nutrition, as does much alternative medicine.

Biopsy: This procedure, often used to diagnose a growth, involves the "removal and examination, usually microscopic, of tissue from the living body." This is generally critical to be able to correctly diagnose cancer.

Cachexia: A condition of physical wasting away and malnutrition, common in cancer patients. It is especially common in humans with pancreatic cancer, which involves rapid weight loss.

Carcinoma: A malignant growth made of epithelial cells that tend to infiltrate the surrounding tissues; it may metastasize.

Complete remission: A tumor can no longer be detected at all.

Cycle: The order or schedule in which chemotherapy drugs are given.

Neoplasm: A type of tumor that contains abnormal cells proliferating in an uncontrolled manner.

Oncology: The medical field that deals with diagnosing and treating cancer. An oncologist is a doctor who specializes in this field. Veterinarians become board-certified in either medical oncology or radiation oncology by completing a residency and passing qualifying examinations.

Palliate: To relieve without curing or mitigating; to alleviate.

Partial remission: A tumor decreases in size by 50 percent or more.

Primary site: The site where the cancerous tumor began.

Prognosis: A forecast; how things look.

Protocol: A specific chemotherapy or overall treatment plan.

Remission: A decrease in a tumor; also, the time when the tumor is smaller.

Sarcoma: A malignant tumor of connective tissue origin (such as bone, muscle, or cartilage).

Notes

Chapter 1: Today's Pets, Today's Cancer

1. Hill's Pet Nutrition Web site, http://www.hillspet.com/index.jsp.
2. *Morris Animal Foundation Animal Health Survey, Fiscal Year 1998,* March 1998, 11.
3. "Be a Guardian," (in an ad, from In Defense of Animals) *Paws to Think* 3, no. 3 (Summer 2004): 20.
4. Stray Rescue/Randy Grim website, "Missouri Recognized Animal Guardians," http://www.strayrescue.org (accessed November 10, 2004).
5. *U.S. Pet Ownership & Demographics Sourcebook,* 2002 edition, http://www.avma.org/membshp/marketstats/sourcebook.asp (accessed October 9, 2004).
6. U.S. Pet Ownership & Demographics Sourcebook Survey, American Veterinary Medical Association Web site, www.avma.org.
7. *U.S. Pet Ownership & Demographics Sourcebook,* 2002 edition, www.avma.org/membshp/marketstats/sourcebook.asp (accessed October 9, 2004).
8. Nancy Peterson, "Holiday Tips for Pet Safety," *Humane Society of the United States News,* 7 December, 1999, hsus-media@hsus.org.
9. Katie Boyle and Desmond Morris, forewords, *A Passion for Dogs: The Dogs Home Battersea* (Newton Abbot, Devon, England: David and Charles Publishers, 1992): 184–85.
10. Canadian Animal Network Web site, www.pawprints.com (accessed September 22, 1999; site now discontinued).
11. Delta Society Web site, "Healthy Reasons to Have a Pet," http://www.deltasociety.org/dsc020.htm.
12. Tufts University Survey, http://www.tufts.edu/vet/cfa/Surveys/pets.html.
13. Rachel Querry, "College Courses on Animal Issues Grow," *Humane Society of the United States News*, 3 December 1999, www.hsus.org.

14. Animal Legal Defense Fund, www.aldf.org (accessed October 12, 2004).

15. "Survey Indicates Studying with Pets Can Improve Students' Grades and SATs," *Pet Product News* (December 1999): 74.

16. Alexandra Zissu, "After the Breakup, Here Comes the Joint-Custody Pet," *New York Times,* 22 August 1999, sec. 9, 1–2.

17. Charles Hirshberg and Susan Watts, "Animal E.R.," *Life* 21 (July 1998): 104–14.

18. American Pet Products Manufacturers Association, *As National Pet Week Approaches, Leading Trade Organization Announces 2004 Industry Study Showing Pet Spending at All Time High*, Press release, April 22, 2004, www.appma.org (accessed November 10, 2004).

19. Rory Carroll, "Italy's Love Affair with Pets Continues," Scripps Howard News Service, 10 January 2000.

20. Royal New South Wales Canine Council Ltd (Australia's AKC), http://www.rnswcc.org.au/ (accessed November 10, 2004).

21. PetNet Web site, "Pet Ownership in Australia," http://www.petnet.com.au/statistics.html.

22. Sarah Hartwell, "Cat Food Around the World," http://www.petpeoplesplace.com/Care/Cats/004/23.htm (accessed October 10, 2004).

23. Kenneth Blank, M.D., and John Han-Chih Chang, M.D., OncoLink Web site, University of Pennsylvania Cancer Center, http://www.oncolink.com/causeprevent.

24. C. A. London and D. M. Vail, in *Clinical Veterinary Oncology*, ed. Stephen J. Withrow and E. G. MacEwen (Philadelphia: Lippincott, 1989).

25. All-Care Animal Referral Center Web site, Animal Health Foundation, Pico Rivera, Calif., http://www.acarc.com.

26. All-Care Animal Referral Center Web site, http://www.acarc.com.

27. Ibid.

28. "Cancer Genetics Program Launched," Yale Cancer Center newsletter, Winter 1996, http://www.info.med.yale.edu.

29. Hill's Pet Nutrition Web site, http://www.hillspet.com/index.jsp.

30. American Veterinary Medical Association Web site, http://www.avma.org/.

31. Ibid.

32. Ibid.

33. University of Pennsylvania Cancer Center, OncoLink Web site "Cancer Terminology and Symptoms," http://www.oncolink.upenn.edu/specialty/ vet_onc (accessed February 14, 1999).

34. Marion S. Lane et al., *Complete Guide to Dog Care, The Humane Society of the United States* (New York: Little, Brown, 1998), 131.

35. Steven E. Crow, D.V.M., "Good Business, Good Medicine," *DVM Web* news magazine, November 1997 http://www.dvmnewsmagazine.com/ sagb9711.html.

36. Ibid.

37. Terri McGinnis, D.V.M., *The Well Dog Book: The Classic Comprehensive Handbook of Dog Care* (New York: Random House, 1991), 214.

38. Amy Marder, "Problem Solvers for Old-Timers," *Prevention* 51, April 1999, 193.

39. Notes from the January 2004 North American Veterinary Conference. *What's*

New in Small Animal Oncology, http://holistic-vet.com/cancer%20integrative.htm (accessed October 16, 2004).

40. Lane et al., *Complete Guide to Dog Care*, 103.

41. Rachel Carson, *Silent Spring* (Boston: Houghton Mifflin, 1962), 241.

42. Ibid., 243.

43. Myrna Milani, D.V.M., e-mail messages to author, October 11–21, 2004.

44. Alfred J. Plechner, D.V.M., and Martin Zucker, *Pets at Risk, From Allergies to Cancer, Remedies for an Unsuspected Epidemic* (Troutdale, Ore: NewSage Press, 2003), ix.

45. Ibid., 71.

46. Ibid., x.

47. Robert McDowell, N.D., *Herbs for Dogs,* http://www.Herbal-DogKeeping.com (accessed November 1, 2004).

48. Robert McDowell, N.D., e-mail message to author, September 3, 2004.

Chapter 2: Dogs

1. Matthew Cravatta, "(Feline) Kings of the Castle," BPD Group's Pet Incidence Trend Report, *American Demographics* 19 (August 1997): 30–31.

2. Susan Milius, "Dogs and Cats in Their Dotage," *Science News* 154 (17 October 1998): 252–54.

3. PetNet Web site, "Pet Ownership in Australia, 2002" http://www.petnet.com.au/statistics.html.

4. Gary J. Patronek, David J. Waters, and Lawrence T. Glickman, "Comparative Longevity of Pet Dogs and Humans: Implications for Gerontology Research," *The Journals of Gerontology, Series A* 52 (May 1997): B171–78.

5. *Poochnooz* 2, no. 10, 20 October 1999, http://www.flintdogfood.com/poochnooz-archives.htm.

6. Melinda Roth, *The Man Who Talks to Dogs . . . The Story of America's Wild Street Dogs and Their Unlikely Savior.* (New York: Thomas Dunne Books, 2002).

7. Nathan B. Sutter and Elaine A. Ostrander, National Human Genome Research Institute, *Dog Star Rising, The Canine Genetic System*, http://www.genome.gov/Pages/About/RecentArticles/OstranderDogViewNatureCommentary.pdf (accessed December 15, 2004).

8. Morris Animal Foundation, "Canine Cancer Facts," *Animal News* 3 (1999): 8.

9. Sutter and Ostrander, *Dog Star Rising, The Canine Genetic System*, http://www.genome.gov/Pages/About/RecentArticles/OstranderDogViewNatureCommentary.pdf.

10. Connie Vanacore, delegate to the American Kennel Club for the Irish Setter Club of America and chairperson of the Health Committee, personal correspondence, January 10, 2000.

11. Frode Lingaas, Kenine E. Comstock, Ewen F. Kirkness, Anita Sorensen, et al., "A mutation in the canine BHD gene is associated with hereditary multifocal renal cystadenocarcinoma and nodular dermatofibrosis in the German Shepherd dog," *Human Molecular Genetics* 12, 23 (2003): 3043–53.

12. Chris C. Pinney, D.V.M., *The Illustrated Veterinary Guide for Dogs, Cats, Birds and Exotic Pets* (New York: TAB Books, McGraw-Hill, 1992), 627.

13. "Oral Melanoma Study: Results to Date Promising," *Canine Times Newsletter* 1, no. 19 (6 December 1997).

14. Norma Bennett Woolf, "Human Cancer Treatment Goes to the Dogs," *Dog Owner's Guide* Web magazine, 1999, http://www.canismajor.com/dog.

15. Tom Ewing, "Skin Cancer: A Common Killer, Owner's Alert: Early Detection of a Malignant Tumor Can Save Your Dog's Life." *Dog Watch* 8, no. 10 (October 2004): 1 and 10.

16. Woolf, "Human Cancer Treatment Goes to the Dogs," http://www.canismajor.com/dog.

17. Mike Richards, D.V.M., Vetinfo Web site, http://www.vetinfo.com/dmelanoma.html.

18. Robert Runyan, D.V.M., "Mammary Tumors are Common, but Declining," *Petview Magazine Online,* National Pet Health and Care Network, 6 December 1999, http://www.petview.com/pc/danemamm.html.

19. Ibid.

20. Woolf, "Human Cancer Treatment Goes to the Dogs," http://www.canismajor.com/dog.

21. Stephen J. Withrow, D.V.M., "Biodegradable Cisplatin Polymer in Limb-Sparing Surgery for Canine Osteosarcoma *"Annals of Surgical Oncology* 2004, http://www.annalssurgicaloncology.org/ (accessed October 17, 2004).

22. Holistic-vet.com, *Lymphoma, Cancer: An Integrative Holistic Approach,* http://holistic-vet.com/cancer%20integrative.htm (accessed October 16, 2004).

23. "Canine Lymphoma: Increasing the Effectiveness of Treatments," *Animal News: Improving the Health and Well-Being of Companion Animals and Wildlife* 3 (1999): 3.

24. Lili Duda, V.M.D., "OncoLink FAQ: Treatment of Canine Lymphoma," University of Pennsylvania Cancer Center, OncoLink Web site, http://www.oncolink.upenn.edu/specialty/vet_onc (accessed August 26, 1999).

25. Gregory Ogilvie, D.V.M., "Canine Cancer Q & A," Morris Animal Foundation Web site, http://www.morrisanimalfoundation.org (accessed April 4, 1997).

26. Pinney, *The Illustrated Veterinary Guide for Dogs, Cats, Birds and Exotic Pets,* 628.

27. Stephen Budiansky, "The Truth About Dogs," *The Atlantic,* (July 1999): 41.

28. Linda Mills, ed., "Endocrine and Metabolic Disorders," in *Kirk's Current Veterinary Therapy XI: Small Animal Practice* (Philadelphia: W. B. Saunders, 1992), 316.

29. Randy Grim, in discussion with the author, September 19, 2004.

30. Ibid.

31. Ed Migneco, D.V.M., in discussion with the author, October 11, 2004.

32. Delbert Carlson, D.V.M., and James Griffin, M.D., *The Dog Owner's Home Veterinary Guide,* Dog Owner's Guide Web magazine, http://www.canismajor.com/dog.

33. Federal Emergency Management Agency, "Canine Search and Rescue Teams'

Response to the 9/11 Attacks," http://www.fema.gov/about/mediacanine.shtm.

34. Cynthia Otto, D.V.M., e-mail message to author, November 4, 2004.

35. Heidi Evans, *New York Daily News,* "14 WTC Search and rescue dogs dead," http://www.nydailynews.com (accessed August 22, 2004).

36. Cynthia Otto, D.V.M., e-mail message to author, November 4, 2004.

37. University of Pennsylvania, *Science Daily,* "9/11 Search-and-rescue Dogs Exhibit Few Effects from Exposure to Disaster Sites," http://www.sciencedaily.com (accessed September 15, 2004).

38. Cynthia Otto, D.V.M., e-mail message to author, November 4, 2004.

39. FDA Center for Veterinary Medicine, *Freedom of Information Summary,— Neutersol,* http://www.fda.gov/cvm/efoi/section2/141-217.pdf (accessed October 19, 2004).

40. Joyce Briggs, "The Spay Shot—a Silver Bullet for Pet Population Control?" *Paws to Think,* vol. 3, no. 4 (Autumn 2004), 15–16.

41. Ed Migneco, D.V.M., e-mail message to author, October 18 , 2004.

42. Mary Elizabeth Thurston, *The Lost History of the Canine Race: Our 15,000-Year Love Affair with Dogs* (Kansas City: Andrews and McMeel, 1996), 120.

43. Mark Derr, "The Politics of Dogs," *The Atlantic* 265 (March 1990): 49–64.

44. Gary F. Mason, "Eliminating Genetic Diseases in Dogs: A Buyer's Perspective," *Working Dogs Cyberzine,* http://www.workingdogs.com/eliminating_gen.htm.

45. Derr, "The Politics of Dogs": 49–64.

46. Mark Derr, "The Perfect Dog," *The Bark* 8 (1999): 32.

47. Dug Hanbicki, interview, December 2, 1999.

48. Robert Johnson, "Sick as a Dog: Pet Stores That Peddle Ailing Canines Face 'Puppy Lemon Laws,'" *Wall Street Journal,* 10 February 1999, 1.

49. Humane Society of the United States, "Get the facts on puppy mills," http://www.hsus.org/Pets/issues-affecting-our-pets (accessed December 30, 2004).

50. Marilyn Putz, e-mail message to author, August 30, 2004.

51. Heidi Jeter, Morris Animal Foundation, e-mail message to author, November 19, 2004.

52. Heidi Jeter, Morris Animal Foundation, e-mail message to author, August 18, 2004.

53. Heidi Jeter, e-mail message to author, August 19, 2004.

54. Rebecca Jones, "Tales of Cancer Survival Unleash Real Job," *Denver Rocky Mountain News,* 9 October 1999.

55. Erika Werne, AKC, e-mail list of cancer grants, sent to author, November 15, 2004.

56. Erika Werne, AKC, e-mail message to author, November 19, 2004.

57. Heidi Parker, e-mail message to author, October 27, 2004.

58. Ibid.

59. *Canine Cancer Awareness, A Guide to Cancer and Mast Cell Tumors in Dogs* (Mendenhall, Pa.: Norwegian Elkhound Rescue, the John Nelsen Moosedog Rescue Fund, 2004), www.elkhoundrescue.org.

60. Sarah Ercolani, e-mail message to author, September 12, 2004.

Chapter 3: Cats

1. Discovery Channel TV, "The Ultimate Guide to House Cats," November 29, 1999.

2. Pet Food Institute statistics, http://www.pfionline.org.

3. Humane Society of the United States, "U.S. Pet Ownership Statistics," www.hsus.org (accessed 1999).

4. Marcus Schneck and Jill Caravan, *Cat Facts* (Rockleigh, N. J.: Barnes and Noble Books, 1993), 11.

5. Cats Protection League Web site, "Cat Facts," http://www.cats.org.uk/ (accessed 1996).

6. BBC News, "World's Oldest Cat Dies," http://news.bbc.co.uk (accessed November 7, 2001).

7. Humane Society of the United States, "Just One Litter . . . Facts About Spaying and Neutering Your Pet," http://www.hsus.org.

8. Ibid.

9. Denise Kessler, D.V.M., personal conversation, February 16, 2000.

10. University of Pennsylvania Cancer Center OncoLink Web site, "Feline Mammary Tumors," www.oncolink.upenn.edu/specialty/vet_onc (accessed February 14, 1999).

11. Lili Duda, V.M.D., "Use of Prednisone in Cats' Cancer Treatment," University of Pennsylvania Cancer Center 25, OncoLink Web site, www.oncolink.upenn.edu/specialty/vet_onc (accessed December 1999).

12. University of Pennsylvania Cancer Center, OncoLink Web site, "Ask Dr. Mike," www.oncolink.upenn.edu/specialty/vet_onc.

13. Ibid.

14. H. Molander-McCrary, C. J. Henry, K. Potter, J. W. Tyler, and M. S. Buss, "Cutaneous Mast Cell Tumors in Cats: 32 Cases (1991–1994)," *Journal of American Animal Hospital Association* 34 (July–August 1998): 281–84.

15. Donna Raditic, D.V.M., personal conversation, June 18, 2000.

16. Amy Marder, V.M.D., "Virus Protection for Your Cat," *Prevention* 47 (March 1995): 126.

17. American Animal Hospital Association Web site "Common Health Problems: Feline Leukemia," http://www.healthypet.com.

18. Anita Frazier with Norma Eckroate, *The New Natural Cat: A Complete Guide for Finicky Owners,* rev. ed. (New York: Dutton/Penguin, 1990), 328.

19. Bree Bisnette, "Cats with Feline Leukemia or FIV (Feline Immunodeficiency Virus) Require Extra Attention," *Kansas State University News,* 13 February 1997, http://www.newss.ksu.edu/WEB/News/NewsReleases/pethealth.html.

20. Jill Roberts-Wilson, D.V.M., *Petview Magazine Online,* National Pet Health and Care Network, www.petview.com/pc/felv.html (accessed December 6, 1999).

21. Richard Pitcairn, D.V.M., and Susan Hubble Pitcairn, *Dr. Pitcairn's Complete Guide to Natural Health for Dogs and Cats,* rev. ed. (Emmaus, Penn.: Rodale Press, 1995), 117, 141.

22. Ibid., 120.

23. Heidi Jeter, e-mail message to author, September 17, 2004.

24. The Winn Feline Foundation, http://www.winnfelinehealth.org/ (accessed September 27, 2004).

25. Susan Little, D.V.M., e-mail message to author, September 17, 2004.

26. Susan Little, D.V.M., e-mail message to author, September 18, 2004.

27. Dale Moss, e-mail message to author, September 16, 2004, used with permission.

Chapter 4: Other Small Animals

1. Canadian Animal Network Web site, "Ferrets," www.pawprints.com (accessed September 22, 1999; site now discontinued).

2. *Morris Animal Foundation Animal Health Survey, Fiscal Year 1998*, March 1998, 11.

3. Canadian Animal Network Web site, www.pawprints.com (accessed September 22, 1999; site now discontinued).

4. Humane Society of the United States, "HSUS Statement on Ferrets as Pets," http://www.hsus.org (accessed October 20, 2004).

5. Alicia Drakiotes, "Ferret Wise," Petsville Library Web site, http://www.petsville.com (accessed July 14, 1998).

6. Susan A. Brown, D.V.M., "Neoplasia," in *Ferrets, Rabbits, and Rodents: Clinical Medicine and Surgery*, eds. Elizabeth V. Hillyer, D.V.M., and Katherine E. Quesenberry, D.V.M. (Philadelphia: W. B. Saunders, 1997), 99.

7. Ibid., 100.

8. Kevin Fitzgerald, D.V.M., *Emergency Vets*, Animal Planet TV, August 5, 1999.

9. Alicia Drakiotes, "Insulinoma in Ferrets," Ferret Wise, Petsville Library Web site, http://www.petsville.com.

10. Mary R. Shefferman, *An Owner's Guide to a Happy Healthy Pet: The Ferret* (New York: Howell Book House, 1996), 86.

11. Drakiotes, "Insulinoma in Ferrets," http://www.petsville.com.

12. Ruth Adams, D.V.M., Ferret Clinic Web site http://www.ferretnews.org:80/lymphosarcoma.html.

13. Elizabeth V. Hillyer, D.V.M., and Katherine E. Quesenberry, D.V.M., eds., *Ferrets, Rabbits, and Rodents: Clinical Medicine and Surgery* (Philadelphia: W. B. Saunders, 1997), 69.

14. Ruth Adams, D.V.M., Ferret Clinic Web site http://www.ferretnews.org:80/lymphosarcoma.html.

15. Thomas J. Burke, "Skin Disorders of Rodents, Rabbits, and Ferrets," *Kirk's Current Veterinary Therapy: Small Animal Practice XI* (Philadelphia: W. B. Saunders, 1992), 1173.

16. Dian Bodofsky, "Herbal Therapy . . . Hope for Our Ferrets," New Rainbow Bridge Web site, http://www.newrainbowbridge.com.

17. Barb Deeb, D.V.M., "Dr. Barb Deeb's Guide to Guinea Pig Care," Allpet Veterinary Clinic Web site, www.halcyon.com/integra/drdeeb.html; (site now discontinued).

18. Holly Mullen, D.V.M., "Soft Tissue Surgery," in Hillyer and Quesenberry, *Ferrets, Rabbits, and Rodents: Clinical Medicine and Surgery*, 287–88.

19. Cavy Care Web site, "Cavy Health Information," http://www.geocities.com/Heartland/Plains/2517.

20. Rebecca Werner, e-mail message to author, February 6, 2004.

21. Humane Society of the United States, "How to Care for Rabbits," www.hsus.org (accessed October 20, 2004).

22. Corrine Fayo, "Rabbit Diseases," http://www.geocities.com/Heartland/Valley/1155/disease.html (accessed 1997).

23. Humane Society of the United States, "How to Care for Rabbits," www.hsus.org (accessed October 20, 2004).

24. Carolina James, "Choosing the Right Type of Litter," Rabbit Charity Web site http://www.therabbitcharity.freeserve.co.uk/index.html.

25. Marinell Harriman, *House Rabbit Handbook: How to Live with an Urban Rabbit* (Alameda, Calif.: Drollery Press 1991), 76.

26. House Rabbit Society Web site, "FAQ: Medical Concerns," http://www. rabbit.org.

27. Joanne Paul-Murphy, D.V.M., "Reproductive and Urogenital Disorders," in Hillyer and Quesenberry, *Ferrets, Rabbits, and Rodents: Clinical Medicine and Surgery,* 202.

28. Cinammon Gimness, *Spaying or Neutering Your Rabbit,* Animal Radio monthly newsletter, August 24, 2004, http://AnimalRadio.com.

29. Linda Dykes and Owen Davies "Uterine Cancer in the Doe: What's the Story?" British Houserabbit Association Web site, http://www.houserabbit.co.uk/.

30. Ibid.

31. Susan A. Brown, D.V.M., "To Neuter or Not to Neuter . . . That Is the Question," Rabbit Charity Web site http://www.therabbitcharity.freeserve.co.uk/neuter.html.

32. Joanne Paul-Murphy, D.V.M., "Reproductive and Urogenital Disorders," 203.

33. Susan A. Brown, D.V.M., "To Neuter or Not to Neuter . . . That is the Question."

34. Ibid.

35. British Houserabbit Association Web site, http://www.houserabbit.co.uk/.

36. British Houserabbit Association Web site, "Having Your Rabbit Neutered," http://www.houserabbit.co.uk/.

37. R. Borkowski and A. Z. Karas, *Clin. Tech. Small Animal Practice* 14 (February 1999): 44–49.

38. Harriman, *House Rabbit Handbook: How to Live with an Urban Rabbit,* 77.

39. Susan A. Brown, D.V.M., "To Neuter or Not to Neuter . . . That Is the Question."

40. Ibid.

Chapter 5: Environmental Concerns

1. National Cancer Institute, Cancer Facts, "Cancer Clusters," January 1999, http://www.cancernet.nci.nih.gov (accessed January 1999).

2. Earl Mindell and Elizabeth Renaghan, *Earl Mindell's Nutrition and Health for Dogs* (Rocklin, Calif.: Prima Publishing, 1998), 85–87.

3. U.S. Environmental Protection Agency, "Indoor Air—Radon," http://www.epa.gov/radon/index.html (accessed October 23, 2004).

4. "The Last Word," *Animal Guardian* magazine, Fall 2003, back cover.

5. American Society for the Prevention of Cruelty to Animals (ASPCA), "Pet Health Alert: Products Sweetened with Xylitol Can Be Toxic to Dogs—News Alert," http://www.news-alert@aspca.org (accessed on August 4, 2004).

6. Dana Farbman, "News Alert, Forbidden Fruit: Grapes and Raisins can be toxic to Dogs," American Society for the Prevention of Cruelty to Animals (ASPCA), http://www.news-alert@aspca.org (accessed July 15, 2004).

7. U.S. Environmental Protection Agency, "Sources of Indoor Air Pollution—Organic Gases (Volatile Organic Compounds—VOCs)," http://www.epa.gov/iaq/voc.html (accessed October 20, 2004).

8. Amy Carlton, "Spring Cleaning: Using Pet-Save Products to Clean Your Home," *Holistic Hound, The Newsletter of Natural Health for Dogs,* 2000.

9. Dana Farbman, American Society for the Prevention of Cruelty to Animals (ASPCA), *News Alert,* http://news-alert@aspca.org (accessed August 26, 2004).

10. Julie Dahlke, D.V.M., "A Pet Owner's Guide to Common Small Animal Poisons," American Veterinary Medical Association Web site, www.avma.org.

11. Steven E. Crow, D.V.M., "Good Business, Good Medicine," *DVM Newsmagazine* http://www.dvmnewsmagazine.com/dvm/.

12. Tom Ewing, "Skin Cancer: A Common Killer, Owner's Alert: Early Detection of a Malignant Tumor Can Save Your Dog's Life," *Dog Watch* (Cornell University College of Veterinary Medicine), (October 2004): 10.

13. Howard M. Hayes, Robert E. Tarone, Kenneth P. Cantor, Carl R. Jessen, Dennis M. McCurnin, and Ralph C. Richardson, "Case-Control Study of Canine Malignant Lymphoma: Positive Association with Dog Owner's Use of 2,4 Dichlorophenoxyacetic Acid Herbicides," *Journal of the National Cancer Institute* 83 (1991): 1226–31.

14. American Veterinary Medical Association, "Herbicide Exposure May Increase Cancer Risk in Dogs," April 15, 2004 press release, http://www.avma.org/press/releases/040415%5Fherbicide%5Fexposure.asp.

15. Theresa A. Fuess, "Cancer Risks in Cats and Dogs," CEPS/Veterinary Extension Web site, http://www.cvm.uiuc.edu/CEPS/PetColumns.cancercb.htm (accessed January 19, 1998).

16. David Hosansky, "Regulating Pesticides," CQ Researcher 9, 29 (August 1999) (online database, http://www.cqpress.com, accessed October 21, 2004).

17. Ibid.

18. PAN Pesticides Database-Pesticide Products, Pesticide Action Network (by S. Orme and S. Kegley), http://www.pesticideinfo.org (accessed October 21, 2004).

19. U.S. Environmental Protection Agency, "Chemicals Evaluated for Carcinogenic Potential," http://www.epa.gov (accessed October 25, 2004).

20. Nina Anderson and Howard Peiper, *Are You Poisoning Your Pets? A Guidebook to How Our Lifestyles Affect the Health of Our Pets* (Garden City Park, N.Y.: Avery Publishing Group, 1998): 64.

21. Defenders of Wildlife, "20 Consumer and Environmental Groups Ask Home Depot and Lowe's to Supply Poison-Free Products for Lawns and Landscapes," April 13, 2005 press release, http://www.defenders.org/releases/pr2005/pr041305.html.

22. "Mortality Study of Golf Course Superintendents," (paper) Golf Course Superintendents Association of America 65th International Golf Course Conference, 1994, http://www.tec.nccnsw.org.au/member/tec/projects/tcye/detail/ CommunitySpaces/golfsups_45.html.

23. Sara Chamberlain, "Golf Endangers Hawai'ian Ecology and Culture," http://www.earthisland.org/journal/golf.html.

24. National Cancer Institute, CancerNet Web site, Cancer Facts, "Environmental Tobacco Smoke," http://www.cancernet.nci.nih.gov (accessed February 1995).

25. Roger Govier, "Chew on This," *The Whole Dog Journal* 2 (August 1999): 11–12.

26. Ibid.

27. "PETsMART Issues Consumer Advisory on Dog Chews," *Pet Product News,* January 2000, 10.

28. "Edward Lowe Brought Cats in from the Cold," *People Weekly* 44, 23 October 1995, 84.

29. Marina Michaels, "Clumping Clay Kitty Litters: A Deadly Convenience," http://www.sonic.net/marina/articles/clump.html.

30. Ibid.

31. Marina Michaels, "Clumping Clay Kitty Litters: Need More Data?" http://www.sonic.net/marina/articles/clump.html.

32. Ibid.

33. Canadian Centre for Occupational Health and Safety (CCOHS) Web site, "Health Effects of Quartz Silica," http://www.ccohs.ca/oshanswers/ chemicals/chem_profiles/quartz_silica/health_qua.html.

34. Frontline Web site, http://www.frontline.com.

35. Cornell University's Pesticide Management Education Program Web site, "Fipronil (Frontline)," http://pmep.cce.cornell.edu/ (accessed March 17, 1998).

36. Terri McGinnis, D.V.M., *The Well Dog Book: The Classic Comprehensive Handbook of Dog Care* (New York: Random House, 1991), 112.

37. Jill A. Richardson, D.V.M., "CFA Health Committee: Cats and Flea Control Products," www.cafinc.org/health.

38. E. Kathryn Meyer, V.M.D., "Cat Owners Beware: Flea Products Labeled for Use Only on Dogs Can Be Fatal to Cats," *JAVMA,* 15 July 1999, The United States Pharmacopoeial Convention, http://www.usp.org.

39. Tom Ellis, "A Flea Pill for Dogs," Michigan State University Extension, Entomology Web site, http://www.msue.msu.edu (accessed September 1, 1999).

40. Donna Raditic, D.V.M., personal conversation, June 18, 2000.

41. Richard H. Pitcairn, D.V.M., and Susan Hubble Pitcairn, *Dr. Pitcairn's Complete Guide to Natural Health for Dogs and Cats,* rev. ed. (Emmaus, Penn.: Rodale Press, 1995): 102–3.

42. Martin Goldstein, D.V.M., *The Nature of Animal Healing: The Path to Your Pet's Health, Happiness, and Longevity* (New York: Alfred A. Knopf, 1999), 216–17.

43. Pat Lazarus, *Keep Your Dog Healthy the Natural Way* (New York: Fawcett Books, 1999), 177.

44. Norine Dworkin, "Naturally Flea-Free," *Vegetarian Times,* September 1998, 18.

45. "How to Keep Your Kids Safe from Pesticides," *Ladies Home Journal,* September 1999, 116.

46. John A. Bukowski and Daniel Wartenberg, "An Alternative Approach for Investigating the Carcinogenicity of Indoor Air Pollution: Pets as Sentinels of Environmental Cancer Risk," *Environmental Health Perspectives* 105 (December 1997): 1312–19.

Chapter 6: Drinking Water

1. Katie Boyle and Desmond Morris, forewords, *A Passion for Dogs: The Dogs Home Battersea* (Newton Abbot, Devon, England: David and Charles Publishers, 1992): 93.

2. David A. Dzanis, D.V.M., "Water: The Forgotten Nutrient," *Catnip,* May 1999, 9.

3. Bruce Fogle, D.V.M., *The Complete Illustrated Guide to Dog Care and Behavior* (San Francisco: Thunder Bay Press, 1999), 175.

4. Steven J. Covert, D.V.M., "Feeding the Dog," University of Missouri-Columbia, agricultural publication G09920, http://www.muextension.missouri.edu/xplor/agguides/pets/g09920.htm (accessed December 9, 1999).

5. Terri McGinnis, D.V.M., *The Well Cat Book: The Classic Comprehensive Handbook of Cat Care* (New York, Random House, 1993), 66.

6. Dzanis, "Water: The Forgotten Nutrient," 9.

7. Pat Lazarus, *Keep Your Dog Healthy the Natural Way* (New York: Fawcett Books, 1999), 53.

8. Eliot Marshall, "The Fluoride Debate: One More Time," *Science* 247 (19 January 1990): 276–77.

9. J. B. Sibbison, "USA: More About Fluoride," *The Lancet* 336 (22 September 1990), 737.

10. Layla Dayani, "Drugs on Tap," *The Ecologist* 33/6 (July/August 2003): 54.

11. British Anti-Vivisection Association, "British New Labour Government 'Health Care': The Corruption Mounts," http://www.bava.pwp.blueyonder.co.uk/labour.html (accessed September 15, 2004).

12. Ahmed Elbetieha, Homa Darmani, Ahmad S. Al-Hiyasat and Jordan Irbid, "Fertility Effects of Sodium Fluoride in Male Mice," *Fluoride* 33/3 (2000): 128–34.

13. Lazarus, *Keep Your Dog Healthy the Natural Way,* 53.

14. Leon Jaroff, "Water Hazard? Finnish Scientists Link Chlorine to Cancer in Rats," *Time* 149, 30 June 1997, 60.

15. "Chlorine: A Special Problem for Drinking Water," Doulton Water Filters H20 International Web site, www.doulton.ca/chlroine.html.

16. Gayle H. Shimokura, David A. Savitz, and Elaine Symanski, "Assessment of Water Use for Estimating Exposure to Tap Water Contaminants," *Environmental Health Perspectives* 106 (February 1998): 55–59.

17. MTBE segment, *60 Minutes,* January 16, 2000.

18. Ibid.

19. Glenn Hess, "EPA Urges a Nationwide Phaseout of MTBE in Reformulated Gasoline," *Chemical Market Report* 256 (2 August 1999): 1.

20. "EPA Plans Ban on Gas Additive," Phillip Brasher, *Burlington Free Press,* 21 March 2000.

21. H. Josef Hebert, "House Votes to Protect Makers of MTBE," *ABC News* 21 April 2005, http://abcnews.go.com/Politics/wireStory?id=691724.

22. Richard H. Pitcairn, D.V.M., and Susan Hubble Pitcairn, *Dr. Pitcairn's Complete Guide to Natural Health for Dogs and Cats,* rev. ed. (Emmaus, Penn.: Rodale Press, 1995), 111–12.

23. Doctors Foster and Smith online catalog, http://www.drsfostersmith.com.

24. Katie Boyle and Desmond Morris, forewords, *A Passion for Dogs: The Dogs Home Battersea,* 50.

25. Lazarus, *Keep Your Dog Healthy the Natural Way,* 54–55.

26. Ibid., 65.

27. Susan W. Putnam and Jonathan Baert Wiener, "Seeking Safe Drinking Water" (Cambridge, Mass.: Harvard University Press, 1995), reprinted on Chlorine Chemistry Council Web site, http://www.c3.org/chlorine_knowledge_center/12749.html.

28. Dzanis, "Water: The Forgotten Nutrient," 10.

Chapter 7: Nutrition

1. "Companion Animal Nutrition: A Survey of Veterinarians," Animal Protection Institute Web site, http://www.api4animals.org (accessed May 30, 2000).

2. Joel Brown and Andi Brown, "Holistic Pet Care," Halo, Purely for Pets (brochure), 2.

3. Ann Martin, *Food Pets Die For: Shocking Facts About Pet Food* (Troutdale, Oreg.: NewSage Press, 1997).

4. Ibid., 25–28.

5. Ibid., 31.

6. Richard H. Pitcairn, D.V.M., and Susan Hubble Pitcairn, *Dr. Pitcairn's Complete Guide to Natural Health for Dogs and Cats,* rev. ed. (Emmaus, Penn.: Rodale Press, 1995), 20.

7. Martin, *Food Pets Die For: Shocking Facts About Pet Food,* 51.

8. Wendell O. Belfield, D.V.M., "Food Not Fit for a Pet," *Your Animal's Health, the Web Magazine for Modern Pet Owners* 3, http://www.belfield.com/article3.html (accessed September 3, 1999).

9. "What Pet Food Labels Tell You," Pet Care Series GP596l, Ralston Purina Company.

10. Tracey C. Rembert, "Natural Critter Care: Rethinking Food, Fun and Fleas for Fido and Fifi," *E: The Environmental Magazine,* May–June 1998.

11. "What's Really in Pet Food?" Animal Protection Institute Web site, http://www.api4animals.org (accessed May 4, 2000).

12. Matthew Cravatta, "(Feline) Kings of the Castle," BPD Group's Pet Incidence Trend Report, *American Demographics* 19 (August 1997): 30–31.

13. "What's Really in Pet Food?" Animal Protection Institute Web site, http://www.api4animals.org (accessed May 4, 2000).

14. June Wholley, "Ethoxyquin: The Tip of the Iceberg," *NaturalPet,* January–February 1994, 22.

15. John Macdonald, "Ethoxyquin," http://www.golden-retriever.com (accessed 1996).

16. Wholley, "Ethoxyquin: The Tip of the Iceberg," 22.

17. "What's Really in Pet Food?" Animal Protection Institute Web site, http://www.api4animals.org (accessed May 4, 2000).

18. Donald R. Strombeck, D.V.M., *Home-Prepared Dog and Cat Diets: The Healthful Alternative* (Ames: Iowa State University Press, 1999), 54–55.

19. Martin, *Food Pets Die For: Shocking Facts About Pet Food,* 92.

20. Narda Robinson, D.V.M., "Complementary Medicine: Test Your Organic Pet Food Savvy," *Veterinary Practice News Online,* http://www.veterinarypractice news.com (accessed October 30, 2004).

21. Martin Goldstein, D.V.M., *The Nature of Animal Healing: The Path to Your Pet's Health, Happiness, and Longevity* (New York: Alfred A Knopf, 1999), 47.

22. Marion S. Lane et al., *Complete Guide to Dog Care, The Humane Society of the United States* (New York: Little, Brown, 1998), 114–15.

23. Ibid., 115–16.

24. "New Holistic Approach to Dog Nutrition," Pet Products Plus Web site, http://www.pppinc.com/holistic.htm (accessed 1996).

25. Narda Robinson, D.V.M., "Complementary Medicine: Test Your Organic Pet Food Savvy," *Veterinary Practice News Online,* http://www.veterinarypractice news.com (accessed October 30, 2004).

26. Steve Brown & Beth Taylor, *See Spot Live Longer: How to Help Your Dog Live a Longer and Healthier Life!* (Eugene, Ore.: Creekobear Press, 2004), preface.

27. Christine McCollum, Natura Pet Products Customer Service, letter to author, July 26, 2004.

28. Donna Raditic, D.V.M., personal conversation, December 21, 1999.

29. Nick Downing, "1999 and Beyond, Trends in Competition, Distribution and New Products," *PetFood Industry* (January–February 1999): 18–19.

30. Ibid.

31. Ibid., 21.

32. Pat Lazarus, *Keep Your Dog Healthy the Natural Way* (New York, Fawcett Books, 1999), 43.

33. Pitcairn and Pitcairn, *Dr. Pitcairn's Complete Guide to Natural Health for Dogs and Cats,* 71–75.

34. Ibid., 71.

35. Ibid., 25–37.

36. Lorelei Wakefield, e-mail message to author, August 30, 2004.

37. Lorelei Wakefield, e-mail message to author, October 11, 2004, and http://www.vegetariancats.com.

38. Donna Raditic, D.V.M., e-mail message to author, November 8, 2004.

39. Catherine O'Driscoll, "Research Proves That Processed Pet Food Is Not Good for Dogs," Canine Health Concern Web site, http://www.canine-health-concern .org.uk/ (accessed August 10, 1996).

40. Dr. Ian Billinghurst, e-mail message to author, December 5, 2004.

41. Robert McDowell, N.D., http://www.herbal-dogkeeping.com (accessed November 2, 2004).

42. Shirley's Wellness Cafe Web site, http://www.shirleys-wellness-cafe.com.

43. Alfred J. Plechner, D.V.M., and Martin Zucker, *Pets at Risk* (Troutdale, Ore.: NewSage Press, 2003), 111.

44. Clare E. Middle, B.V.M.S., personal correspondence, November 3, 1999.

45. Carolyn J. Ashton, B.V.Sc., personal correspondence, January 15, 2000.

46. Kymythy Schultze, "Building a Good Foundation . . . Naturally," Sirius Dog, For the Performance Dog Enthusiast Web site, http://siriusdog.com/articles/index.php.

47. Joe Bodewes, D.V.M., "Homemade Diets," Doctors Foster and Smith Web site, http://www.PetEducation.com.

48. Anita Frazier with Norma Eckroate, *The New Natural Cat: A Complete Guide for Finicky Owners,* rev. ed. (New York: Dutton/Penguin, 1990), 69–70.

49. Sharon Machlik, "Raw Risks: Raw-Food Diets for Dogs Are Difficult and Hazardous," *Petfood Industry* (May–June 1999), 56–57.

50. Dale Moss, "Treating Uly for Cancer," *Yankee Dog 5,* no. 1 (Summer 2004), used with permission.

51. Joseph Hahn, "Don't Feed Your Cat That Dog Food," University of Illinois College of Veterinary Medicine Web site, www.cvm.uiuc.edu/ceps/PetColumns/ catnut.htm (accessed October 14, 1996).

52. "What All Cats Need," *Catnip,* August 1997, 5.

53. "Cooking for Your Cat?" *Catnip,* April 1998, 3.

54. Connolly Animal Clinic, Nacogdoches, TX, "Why is tuna fish bad for cats?" http://www.connollyac.com (accessed November 7, 2004).

55. Frazier with Eckroate, *The New Natural Cat: A Complete Guide for Finicky Owners,* 47–53, 66–67.

56. Alfred J. Plechner, D.V.M., and Martin Zucker, *Pets at Risk, From Allergies to Cancer, Remedies for an Unsuspected Epidemic* (Troutdale, Ore.: NewSage Press, 2003), 60.

57. Bodewes, "Homemade Diets," Doctors Foster and Smith Web site http://www .PetEducation.com.

58. Kathleen Griffin, D.V.M., N.D., from a story by Daska Saleeba, personal correspondence, February 8, 2000.

Chapter 8: Vaccinations

1. W. Jean Dodds, D.V.M., "Changing Vaccine Protocols" appeared in *Veterinary Medicine* 2002, also available at http://www.canine-epilepsy-guardian-angels .com/chang_vac.htm (accessed November 8, 2004).

2. Dana Cox, "Overvaccinated?" *Animal Wellness Magazine* 6, no. 4, 2004, 26.

3. Richard Pitcairn, D.V.M., and Susan Hubble Pitcairn, *Dr. Pitcairn's Complete*

Guide to Natural Health for Dogs and Cats, rev. ed. (Emmaus, Penn.: Rodale Press, 1995), 247.

4. Ibid., 244.

5. Ibid., 324–25.

6. W. Jean Dodds, D.V.M., e-mail message to author, November 9, 2004.

7. Christina Chambreau, D.V.M., "Integrating Homeopathy and Holistic Medicine into Your Veterinary Practice" (lecture), Shirley's Wellness Cafe Web site, http://www.shirleys-wellness-cafe.com/petvaccchambreau.htm.

8. Gary D. Norsworthy, D.V.M., "Another Perspective on the Vaccination Controversy: Proposed Changes in the Standard Feline Vaccination Protocol," *Veterinary Medicine* (August 1999): 731.

9. "US—Vaccine Notification Law Defeated," Brakke Consulting Animal Health News & Notes, April 22, 2005, http://www.brakkeconsulting.com.

10. "Sleuthing Feline Sarcoma," www.wizard.net/~peacock/sleuth.htm (accessed October 28, 1999; site now discontinued).

11. George Glanzberg, V.M.D., personal correspondence, March 5, 2000.

12. "Preventive Care: Vaccine-Associated Feline Sarcoma Task Force," American Animal Hospital Association Web site, http://www.healthypet.com.

13. "Dear Kitty," *CATS Magazine* Web site, http://www.catsmag.com/Pages/dearkitty.html (site now discontinued).

14. Gary D. Norsworthy, D.V.M., "Another Perspective on the Vaccination Controversy," 729.

15. Amy Marder, V.M.D., "The Scoop on Cat Vaccines," *Prevention* 49, March 1997, 143–45.

16. "Sleuthing Feline Sarcoma" http://www.wizard.net/~peacock/sleuth.htm (site now discontinued).

17. Ibid.

18. Vaccine-Associated Feline Sarcoma Task Force of the American Veterinary Medical Association, http://www.avma.org/vafstf (accessed November 4, 2004).

19. Ibid.

20. Tom Elston, D.V.M., phone interview, January 13, 2005.

21. Ibid.

22. M. Vascellari, E. Melchiotti, M. A. Bozza, and F. Mutinelli, "Fibrosarcomas at Presumed Sites of Injection in Dogs: Characteristics and Comparison with Non-vaccination Site Fibrosarcomas and Feline Post-vaccinal Fibrosarcomas," *The Journal of Veterinary Medicine,* (2003): 286–91. http://www.bris.ac.uk/Depts/PathAndMicro/EuroVet/jva_50_286_291.pdf.

23. The American Animal Hospital Association, *Report of the American Animal Hospital Association Canine Vaccine Task Force: 2003 Canine Vaccine Guidelines, Recommendations, and Supporting Literature,* received and cited November 2004.

24. Ibid.

25. Christina Chambreau, D.V.M., "Integrating Homeopathy and Holistic Medicine into Your Veterinary Practice," Shirley's Wellness Cafe Web site,

http://www.shirleys-wellness-cafe.com/petvaccchambreau.htm.

26. Catherine O'Driscoll, "Pet Vaccine Myths," Canine Health Concern Web site, http://www.canine-health-concern.org.uk/.

27. Jane Bicks, D.V.M., "Feline Vaccinations: What's the Story?" *The Pet Tribune On-Line,* http://www.thepettribune.com/1997/111297/32.html.

28. W. Jean Dodds, D.V.M., e-mail message to author, November 8, 2004.

29. W. Jean Dodds, D.V.M., e-mail message to author, November 9, 2004.

30. W. Jean Dodds, D.V.M., and Lisa Twark, D.V.M., "Vaccine Titers in Dogs to Assess Humoral Immune Memory," *Proceedings of the 1999 American Holistic Veterinary Medical Association Annual Conference,* 83–84.

31. W. Jean Dodds, D.V.M., e-mail message to author, November 8, 2004.

32. Goldstein, *The Nature of Animal Healing: The Path to Your Pet's Health, Happiness, and Longevity,* 142–43.

33. Laura Wallingford, "Vaccinosis: Dr. Richard Pitcairn Discusses Chronic Disease Caused by Vaccines," *Wolf Clan Magazine,* 1995, reprinted on Shirley's Wellness Cafe Web site, http://www.shirleys-wellness-cafe.com/vaccines.htm.

34. Ibid.

Chapter 9: The Role of Emotions

1. Gary Kowalski, *The Souls of Animals,* rev. ed. (Walpole, N.H.: Stillpoint Publishing, 1999), 19.

2. Ibid., 122.

3. Ibid., 139.

4. Jane Goodall with Phillip Berman, *Reason for Hope* (New York: Warner Books, 1999), 77–78.

5. Myrna M. Milani, D.V.M., *The Art of Veterinary Practice: A Guide to Client Communication* (Philadelphia: University of Pennsylvania Press, 1995), 70.

6. Ibid., 76.

7. Ibid., 7.

8. Myrna M. Milani, D.V.M., personal correspondence, November 16, 1999.

9. Donna Raditic, D.V.M., personal conversation, December 21, 1999.

10. Molly Sheehan, Green Hope Farm, e-mail messages to author, September 9 & 13, 2004.

11. Darren Hawks, D.V.M., "Your Pet's Health: The Big Picture of the Holistic Approach," http://www.jps.net/dhawks.HA.html (site now discontinued).

12. Betsy Adams, "The Animal/Human Energy Bond," *Sowell Review* (September–October 1999).

13. *Best in Show,* VHS, directed by Christopher Guest, produced by Karen Murphy (Warner Studios, 2000).

14. Samantha Mooney, *A Snowflake in My Hand* (New York: Delacorte Press, 1983), 80.

15. Donna Raditic, D.V.M., personal conversation, December 21, 1999.

16. Milani, *The Art of Veterinary Practice: A Guide to Client Communication,* 197.

17. Sylvia Wright, "Veterinary Ethics Professor Talks About Dilemmas in Human-

Animal Relations," *Canine Times* 86, no. 4, February 3, 2000, http://www
.cfnaonline.com/caninetimes.

18.   Earl Mindell and Elizabeth Renaghan, *Earl Mindell's Nutrition and Health for
Dogs* (Rocklin, Calif.: Prima Publishing, 1998), 79–81.

19.   Anita Frazier with Norma Eckroate, *The New Natural Cat: A Complete Guide
for Finicky Owners,* rev. ed. (New York: Dutton/Penguin, 1990), 198.

20.   Ibid., 200–201.

21.   Kathleen Griffin, D.V.M., N.D., personal correspondence, January 29, 2000.

22.   Kathleen Griffin, D.V.M., N.D., personal correspondence, February 7, 2000.

23.   Peter Barry Chowka, "Prayer Is Good Medicine: An Interview with Larry Dossey,
M.D.," *Yoga Journal* 129, July–August 1996, 60–67, 156–58.

24.   Richard H. Pitcairn, D.V.M., and Susan Hubble Pitcairn, *Dr. Pitcairn's Complete
Guide to Natural Health for Dogs and Cats,* rev. ed. (Emmaus, Penn.: Rodale
Press, 1995), 147–48.

25.   Anna Guitton, D.V.M., personal correspondence, February 4, 2000.

26.   Carolyn J. Ashton, B.V.Sc., personal correspondence, November 2, 1999.

27.   George Glanzberg, V.M.D., personal correspondence, February 3, 2000.

28.   Rita Reynolds, personal correspondence, December 9, 1999.

29.   Milani, *The Art of Veterinary Practice: A Guide to Client Communication,*
215–16.

Chapter 10: Conventional Treatments

1.   "Cancer: Facts Not Fears," *Catnip,* February 1995, 6.

2.   Samantha Mooney, *A Snowflake in My Hand* (New York: Delacorte Press, 1983),
24.

3.   Myrna Milani, D.V.M., e-mail message to author, October 11, 2004.

4.   Holistic-vet.com, *Cancer: An Integrative Holistic Approach,* http://holisticvet
.com/cancer%20integrative.htm (accessed October 17, 2004).

5.   "Multimodality Therapy: Using the Best Available Treatments Together
Rationally," *Canine Cancer: Management of Canine Cancer* (monograph), (Hill's
Prescription Diet, 1998): 44.

6.   Walter Last, "The Diversity and Effectiveness of Natural Cancer Cures," *The
Ecologist* 28 (March–April 1998): 117–21.

7.   Donna Raditic, D.V.M., personal correspondence, January 1, 2000.

8.   "Anesthesia and the Older Cat," *Catnip,* August 1994, 5.

9.   "Anesthesia: Your Cat's Friend," *Catnip,* January 1998, 4.

10.   Sharon Haddock, "Laser Surgery More Pet-Friendly," 27 April 1999,
http://www.deseretnews.com.

11.   "Laser Surgery," *Catnip,* August 1998, 7.

12.   Sharon Haddock, "Laser Surgery More Pet-Friendly," http://www.deseret
news.com.

13.   Ed Garsten, "Drug-Laser Therapy Is Promising Treatment for Pet Cancer," Cable
News Network, 30 August 1996, www.cnn.com.

14.   Donald E. Thrall, "Strategies to Enhance Tumor Radioresponsiveness," *Kirk's*

Current Veterinary Therapy XI: Small Animal Practice (Philadelphia: W. B. Saunders, 1992), 425.

15. Last, "The Diversity and Effectiveness of Natural Cancer Cures," 117–21.

16. Michael Walker, D.V.M., "Veterinary Radiation Oncology," *Veterinary Medicine* (April 1997): 351.

17. Ibid., 356.

18. Ibid., 358.

19. All-Care Animal Referral Center Web site, Animal Health Foundation, Pico Rivera, Calif., http://www.acarc.com.

20. "Radioactive Beads Latest Tool in Fighting Cancer," *DVM* 30 (March 1999): 11S.

21. Ibid.

22. Tomotherapy at the University of Wisconsin-Madison, http:www.psl.wisc.edu/tomo.html (accessed October 29, 2004).

23. Ilene Kurzman ACT, e-mail message to author, October 29, 2004.

24. University of Pennsylvania Cancer Center, "Veterinary Cancer Treatment Options," OncoLink Web site, http://www.oncolink.upenn.edu/specialty/vet_onc/treat/ (accessed April 4, 1997).

25. Last, "The Diversity and Effectiveness of Natural Cancer Cures," 117–21.

26. University of Pennsylvania Cancer Center, "Veterinary Cancer Treatment Options," OncoLink Web site, http://www.oncolink.upenn.edu/specialty/vet_onc/treat/ (accessed April 4, 1997).

27. All-Care Animal Referral Center Web site, http://www.acarc.com/ cancer.html.

28. "Treatment of Cancer in Veterinary Medicine (brochure)," Veterinary Pet Insurance.

29. All-Care Animal Referral Center Web site, http://www.acarc.com.

30. Earl Mindell and Elizabeth Renaghan, *Earl Mindell's Nutrition and Health for Dogs* (Rocklin, Calif.: Prima Publishing, 1998), 133.

31. Christine A. Verstraete, "Something to Bark About—Canine Cancer," *DogWorld,* October 1998, 70.

32. Donna Raditic, D.V.M., personal conversation, February 2000.

33. Denise Kessler, D.V.M., personal conversation, February 2000.

34. MarVista Animal Medical Center and Pharmacy, "Prednisone," http://www.marvistavet.com/html/prednisone.html (accessed October 20, 2004).

35. Myrna Milani, D.V.M., e-mail message to author, October 25, 2004.

36. National Cancer Institute Web site, "Angiogenesis Inhibitors in Cancer Research," Cancer Trials: News and Features, http://www.nih.gov/news/pr/july98/nci-07.htm (accessed March 31, 1999).

37. National Cancer Institute, "Angiogenesis Inhibitors in the Treatment of Cancer," http://cis.nci.nih.gov/fact/7_42.htm (accessed July 9, 1998).

38. University of Wisconsin-Madison School of Veterinary Medicine, *On Call* newsletter, July 2004, http://www2.vetmed.wisc.edu/oncall/about.php (accessed October 15, 2004).

39. Kenneth Marcella, D.V.M., "Transfer Factor: Long-awaited next step in immunotherapy," *DVM Newsmagazine* (February 2003), http://www.dvmnews.com/dvm/article/articleDetail.jsp?id=46984.

40. Shirley Lipschutz-Robinson, Shirley's Wellness Cafe, "Application of Transfer Factor in Veterinary Medicine," http://www.tfpets.com.

41. *Kirk's Current Veterinary Therapy XI: Small Animal Practice,* 416–18.

42. *Kirk's Current Veterinary Therapy XI: Small Animal Practice,* 416.

43. Jim Wilson, "Throwing a Wrench at Cancer," *Popular Mechanics* 176, June 1999, 38.

44. Duke K. Bahn, M.D., "Cryosurgery in the Treatment of Prostate Cancer," *Cancer News,* 1996, 1997, www.cancernews.com.

45. Martin Goldstein, D.V.M., *The Nature of Animal Healing: The Path to Your Pet's Health, Happiness, and Longevity* (New York: Alfred A. Knopf, 1999), 257–65.

46. Ilene Kurzman, ACT Program, e-mail message to author, November 1, 2004.

47. Ibid.

48. Ilene Kurzman, ACT program, e-mail message to author, November 12, 2004.

49. University of Wisconsin-Madison School of Veterinary Medicine, http://www2.vetmed.wisc.edu (accessed October 15, 2004).

50. Richard H. Pitcairn, D.V.M., and Susan Hubble Pitcairn, *Dr. Pitcairn's Complete Guide to Natural Health for Dogs and Cats,* rev. ed. (Emmaus, Penn.: Rodale Press, 1995), 247.

51. Andrew Weil, M.D., "Ask Dr. Weil," www.altmedicine.com (accessed November 18, 1999).

52. Pitcairn and Pitcairn, *Dr. Pitcairn's Complete Guide to Natural Health for Dogs and Cats,* 247.

53. R. M. Clemmons, D.V.M., "Integrative Treatment of Cancer in Dogs," http://neuro.vetmed.ufl.edu/neuro/AltMed/Cancer/Cancer_AltMed.htm.

54. Ibid.

Chapter 11: An Introduction to Alternative Therapies

1. Myrna M. Milani, D.V.M., *The Art of Veterinary Practice: A Guide to Client Communication* (Philadelphia: University of Pennsylvania Press, 1995), 170.

2. Myrna Milani, D.V.M., e-mail message to author, October 11, 2004.

3. Martin Goldstein, D.V.M., *The Nature of Animal Healing, The Path to Your Pet's Health, Happiness, and Longevity* (New York: Alfred A. Knopf, 1999), 298.

4. Jacqueline Stenson, "Alternative Vets Ease Pets' Pain—Americans Seek Holistic Care for Their Animals, Too," *Animal News* 1998, http://www.holisticvets.com/kudos_files/kudon_animalnews.htm.

5. Theresa M. Mall, AHVMA, e-mail message to author, October 11, 2004.

6. Edward C. Boldt Jr., D.V.M., personal correspondence, November 1, 2004.

7. Milani, *The Art of Veterinary Practice: A Guide to Client Communication,* 175.

8. Ibid., 177.

9. Ibid., 178–79.

10. Jacqueline Stenson, "Alternative Vets Ease Pets' Pain," http://www.holisticvets.com/kudos_files/kudon_animalnews.htm.

11. "Guidelines for Alternative and Complementary Veterinary Medicine, Approved by AVMA House of Delegates, 1996," *JAVMA* 209, http://www

.naturalholistic.com/handouts/avmarule.htm (accessed September 15, 1996).

12. AltVetMed Web site, "Visitors to AltVetMed," www.altvetmed.org (accessed 1997).

13. Jan A. Bergeron, V.M.D., personal correspondence, January 2, 2000.

14. "Total Cancer Management in Small Animals," www.altvetmed.org.

15. Holistic-vet.com, from Notes from the 2004 North American Veterinary Conference, from *Manual of Natural Veterinary Medicine: Science and Tradition* by Susan G. Wynn, http://holistic-vet.com/cancer%20integrative.htm (accessed October 16, 2004).

Chapter 12: Herbs and Bach Flower Remedies

1. Susan G. Wynn, D.V.M., "Herbs in Veterinary Medicine," AltVetMed Web site http://www.altvetmed.org.

2. Christine Gorman, "St. Bernard's Wort: Alternative Medicine for Dogs, Cats and Cockatoos: Well, Yes—More and More Americans Believe in It," *Time* 150, 3 November 1997, 93–94.

3. Katie Boyle and Desmond Morris, forewords, *A Passion for Dogs: The Dogs Home Battersea* (Newton Abbot, Devon, England: David and Charles Publishers, 1992), 189–90.

4. Wynn, "Herbs in Veterinary Medicine."

5. Richard H. Pitcairn, D.V.M., and Susan Hubble Pitcairn, *Dr. Pitcairn's Complete Guide to Natural Health for Dogs and Cats,* rev. ed. (Emmaus, Penn.: Rodale Press, 1995), 196–97.

6. Veterinary Botanical Medicine Association, *Herbs for Animals,* http://www.vbma.org (accessed October 25, 2004).

7. Robert McDowell, *The Rise of Canine Cancers,* http://www.herbal-dog keeping.com/article_theriseof_canine_cancers.htm (accessed November 2, 2004).

8. Narda Robinson, D.O., D.V.M., "Treatment Covers Malaria and Cancer," *Veterinary Practice News* 16, no. 9 (September 2004): 36–37.

9. Cancer Information and Support International, http://www.cancer-info.com.

10. Russell Swift, D.V.M., "The Facts About Essiac," *The Pet Tribune On-Line,* http://www.thepettribune.com/1998/020398/22.html.

11. Walter Last, "The Diversity and Effectiveness of Natural Cancer Cures," *The Ecologist* 28 (March–April 1998): 117–21.

12. Pat Lazarus, *Keep Your Dog Healthy the Natural Way* (New York: Fawcett Books, 1999), 215.

13. Clare E. Middle, B.V.M.S., personal correspondence, December 23, 1999.

14. Clare E. Middle, B.V.M.S., "The Use of Essiac in the Treatment of Cancer as an Alternative to Chemotherapy in Small Animal Veterinary Practice" (paper), Australian Veterinary Association Conference, 1996.

15. Elaine Crews, N.D., "Garlic: Nature's Wonder Drug," *The Pet Tribune On-Line,* http://www.thepettribune.com/1998/060798/11.html.

16. Braddock Ray, "Cancer-Fighting Botanicals," *Taste for Life,* Herbal Life Section, October 1999.

17. Last, "The Diversity and Effectiveness of Natural Cancer Cures," 117–21.

18. Elaine Crews, "Garlic: Nature's Wonder Drug," *The Pet Tribune On-Line,* http://www.thepettribune.com/1998/060798/11.html.

19. "Raw Garlic Tackles Cancer," BBC Online Network Web site, http://www.altmedicine.com (accessed June 25, 1999).

20. Lazarus, *Keep Your Dog Healthy the Natural Way,* 278.

21. Patricia Ward Spain, "History of Hoxsey Treatment," www.tldp.com/issue/166/166hoxs.htm.

22. Ibid.

23. Ibid.

24. "Bio-Medical Center, Hoxsey Therapy," Health Resource Web site, http://www.healthworld.com/library/articles/canclinc/hoxsey.htm.

25. Ibid.

26. Spain, "History of Hoxsey Treatment," www.tldp.com/issue/166/166hoxs.htm.

27. Andrew Weil, M.D., "Ask Dr. Weil: New Weapons to Fight Cancer," http://www.pathfinder.com/drweil (accessed November 18, 1999).

28. Kenny Ausubel, personal correspondence, January 13, 2000.

29. Russell Swift, D.V.M., "Milk Thistle: Herbal Wonders," *The Pet Tribune On-Line,* http://www.thepettribune.com/1998/040598/9.html.

30. R. M. Clemmons, D.V.M., "Integrative Treatment of Cancer in Dogs," http://neuro.vetmed.ufl.edu/neuro/AltMed/Cancer/Cancer_AltMed.htm.

31. Pitcairn and Pitcairn, *Dr. Pitcairn's Complete Guide to Natural Health for Dogs and Cats,* 247, 346–47.

32. Sally Deneen, "Stalking Medicinal Plants," *E: The Environmental Magazine* 10, July–August 1999, 39.

33. Becky Gillette, "The Cold War," *E: The Environmental Magazine* 10, January–February 1999, 42–43.

34. Avena Botanicals Herbal Apothecary 1999–2000 catalog, 25.

35. Pitcairn and Pitcairn, *Dr. Pitcairn's Complete Guide to Natural Health for Dogs and Cats,* 87–88.

36. Gregory L. Tilford and Mary Wulff-Tilford, "Top 10 Herbs for Cats: The Best Herbs to Have on Hand," *1999 Annual Natural Cat, Your Complete Guide to Holistic Cat Care* (Fancy Publications, Inc.), 25–26.

37. Ibid.

38. *B-Naturals Newsletter,* Summer 1998, http://b-naturals.com/Sum1998.php.

39. Clemmons, D.V.M., "Integrative Treatment of Cancer in Dogs," http://neuro.vetmed.ufl.edu/neuro/AltMed/Cancer/Cancer_AltMed.htm.

40. Lisa Ayala, NSP Herbs for Pets (brochure).

41. David McCluggage, D.V.M., "An Introduction to Clinical Nutrition: Healing with Nutrition," in *Proceedings of the 1996 American Holistic Veterinary Medical Association Annual Conference,* 23.

42. Clemmons, D.V.M., "Integrative Treatment of Cancer in Dogs," http://neuro.vetmed.ufl.edu/neuro/AltMed/Cancer/Cancer_AltMed.htm.

43. Martin Goldstein, D.V.M., *The Nature of Animal Healing: The Path to Your Pet's*

Health, Happiness, and Longevity (New York: Alfred A. Knopf, 1997), 146–47.

44. "Aloe Vera," http://www.betterlivinguse.com/aloevera.htm.

45. "Aloegold R," *Journal of Ethnopharmacology* 1986, http://www.netunlimited .net/~wcr/aloegold.html.

46. "Aloe Vera: Nothing Beats It," *Canine Times* Web site, 8 September 1999, http://www.cfnaonline.com/caninetimes/topics/cancer.html.

47. Cheryl Schwartz, D.V.M., *Four Paws Five Directions: A Guide to Chinese Medicine for Cats and Dogs* (Berkeley, Calif.: Celestial Arts, 1996), 71.

48. Ibid.

49. Ken Babal, C.N., "The Cancer-Fighting Qualities of Mushrooms," *Nutrition Science News,* March 1997.

50. Karen S. Vaughan, "Re: Reishi Mushrooms," 29 December 1997, http://www.medicinegarden.com.

51. Ibid.

52. Clemmons, D.V.M., "Integrative Treatment of Cancer in Dogs," http://neuro .vetmed.ufl.edu/neuro/AltMed/Cancer/Cancer_AltMed.htm.

53. Russell Swift, D.V.M., "Some Thoughts on Cancer—Holistic Style," *The Pet Tribune On-Line,* November–December 1999, http://www.thepettribune .com/1999/110199/holistic.html.

54. Donna Raditic, D.V.M., personal conversation, June 18, 2000.

55. Clare E. Middle, B.V.M.S., "The Holistic Treatment of Cancer," personal correspondence, November 3, 1999.

56. Clare E. Middle, B.V.M.S., "The Use of Essiac in the Treatment of Cancer as an Alternative to Chemotherapy in Small Animal Veterinary Practice," personal correspondence, November 3, 1999.

57. Carolyn J. Ashton, B.V.M.S., personal correspondence, November 1999.

58. Clare E. Middle, B.V.M.S., personal correspondence, November 3, 1999.

59. Sally Eauclaire Osborne, "Winter Stress Relief: The Calming Benefits of Flower Essences Work for Pets, Too," *Taste for Life,* January 2000.

60. Anita Frazier with Norma Eckroate, *The New Natural Cat: A Complete Guide for Finicky Owners,* rev. ed. (New York: Dutton/Penguin, 1990), 249–51.

61. Rita Reynolds, e-mail message to author, August 4, 2004.

62. Molly Sheehan, *A Guide to Green Hope Farm Flower Essences,* "The Beloved Animals,"(2003), 29.

63. Molly Sheehan, e-mail message to author, August 30, 2004.

Chapter 13: Vitamins and More

1. Catherine O'Driscoll, "Help Your Dog to Stay Young and Beautiful," Canine Health Concern Web site, http://www.canine-health-concern.org.uk/.

2. Lawrence J. Machlin, "Antioxidant Vitamins, Role in Disease Prevention," *PetFood Industry* (November 1993): 11, 38.

3. Pat Lazarus, *Keep Your Dog Healthy the Natural Way* (New York: Fawcett Books, 1999), 274.

4. Catherine O'Driscoll, Canine Health Concern Web site, http://www .canine-health-concern.org.uk/.

5. Ann Martin, *Food Pets Die For: Shocking Facts About Pet Food* (Troutdale Oreg.: NewSage Press, 1997), 100.

6. Richard H. Pitcairn, D.V.M., and Susan Hubble Pitcairn, *Dr. Pitcairn's Complete Guide to Natural Health for Dogs and Cats,* rev. ed. (Emmaus, Penn.: Rodale Press, 1995), 111.

7. Earl Mindell and Elizabeth Renaghan, *Earl Mindell's Nutrition and Health for Dogs* (Rocklin, Calif.: Prima Publishing, 1998), 133.

8. Peter Barry Chowka, "Linus Pauling, Ph.D.: The Last Interview," *Nutrition Science News* 1 (April 1996): 26–28.

9. Mindell and Renaghan, *Earl Mindell's Nutrition and Health for Dogs,* 133.

10. Liz Palika, "Natural Nutrition, 'Oh, Say Can You C?' Learn All About Vitamin C," *1999 Annual Natural Cat, Your Complete Guide to Holistic Cat Care,* 67.

11. "Nutrients: Building Blocks of Canine Fitness," *Dog Owner's Guide* Web magazine, http://www.canismajor.com/dog/nutrit2.html.

12. Martin, *Food Pets Die For: Shocking Facts About Pet Food,* 101.

13. Pitcairn and Pitcairn, *Dr. Pitcairn's Complete Guide to Natural Health for Dogs and Cats,* 76.

14. Machlin, "Antioxidant Vitamins, Role in Disease Prevention," 4, 13–14.

15. Martin, *Food Pets Die For: Shocking Facts About Pet Food,* 114–16.

16. Mindell and Renaghan, *Earl Mindell's Nutrition and Health for Dogs,* 29–30.

17. Kathleen Cheeseman, "Is Vitamin A Toxicity a Real Threat? Or Just an Urban Myth?" League of Independent Ferret Enthusiasts Web site, Ferret Information Bank, (site now discontinued).

18. Robert McDowell, *The Rise of Canine Cancers,* http://www.herbal-dogkeeping .com/article_theriseof_canine_cancers.htm (accessed November 2, 2004).

19. Ibid.

20. Lazarus, *Keep Your Dog Healthy the Natural Way,* 274.

21. Pitcairn and Pitcairn, *Dr. Pitcairn's Complete Guide to Natural Health for Dogs and Cats,* 34–35.

22. Mindell and Renaghan, *Earl Mindell's Nutrition and Health for Dogs,* 44.

23. Machlin, "Antioxidant Vitamins, Role in Disease Prevention," 10–11.

24. Mindell and Renaghan, *Earl Mindell's Nutrition and Health for Dogs,* 134.

25. Drugstore.com Web site, articles, "Selenium," http://www.drugstore.com.

26. Ming-Whei Yu, Ing-Sheng Horng, et al., "Plasma Selenium Levels and Risk of Hepatocellular Carcinoma Among Men with Chronic Hepatitis Virus Infection," *American Journal of Epidemiology* 150, no. 4 (15 August 1999): 367–74.

27. Joel Wallach, D.V.M., http://www.costarr.com/ult_selenium.htm.

28. Lazarus, *Keep Your Dog Healthy the Natural Way,* 278.

29. Susan G. Wynn, D.V.M., "Total Cancer Management in Small Animals," AltVetMed Web site http://www.altvetmed.org.

30. Larry C. Clark et al., "Selenium and Cancer Prevention," *Journal of the American Medical Association* 276 (1996): 1957–63.

31. Wynn, "Total Cancer Management in Small Animals," AltVetMed Web site, http://www.altvetmed.org.

Chapter 14: Homeopathy and Naturopathy

1. Kaetheryn Walker, *Homeopathic First Aid for Animals: Tales and Techniques from a Country Practitioner* (Rochester, Vt.: Healing Arts Press, 1998), 2.

2. Richard Pitcairn, D.V.M., personal correspondence, October 1999.

3. Russell Swift, D.V.M., "Some Thoughts on Cancer—Holistic Style," *The Pet Tribune On-Line,* http://www.thepettribune.com/1999/110199/holistic.html.

4. George Glanzberg, V.M.D., "Complementary Medicine for Pets: The Best of Both Worlds," *Healing Options,* Fall 1999, 7.

5. Ibid.

6. Ibid.

7. Clare E. Middle, D.V.M., "The Holistic Treatment of Cancer," personal correspondence, November 3, 1999.

8. Kathleen Griffin, N.D., personal correspondence, February 7, 2000.

9. Ibid.

10. Carolyn J. Ashton, B.V.Sc., personal correspondence, November 2, 1999.

11. Anna Guitton, D.V.M., personal correspondence, February 2000.

12. General Council and Register of Naturopaths, Naturopathic Medicine in the UK, Definition and Philosophy of Naturopathy, http://www.naturopathy.org.uk/.

13. Natural Therapy Centre for Animals, "Animal Naturopathy," http://www.natural animals.com.au/anmlnat.htm.

14. Killarney Cat Hospital Web site, http://www.catdoctor.ca/.

15. Richard H. Pitcairn, D.V.M., and Susan Hubble Pitcairn, *Dr. Pitcairn's Complete Guide to Natural Health for Dogs and Cats,* rev. ed. (Emmaus, Penn.: Rodale Press, 1995), 195.

16. Kathleen Griffin, N.D., personal correspondence, February 2000.

17. Pitcairn and Pitcairn, *Dr. Pitcairn's Complete Guide to Natural Health for Dogs and Cats,* 295.

18. HomeVet Web site, "Case History: A Natural Diet Restores a Miserably Ill Cat," http://www.homevet.com/index.html (accessed December 18, 1997).

19. Cara Courage, marketing manager, Denes Natural Pet Care Limited, personal correspondence, January 27, 2000.

20. Buster Lloyd-Jones, *Come into My World* (London: Martin Secker and Warburg, 1972), 152.

21. Ibid.

22. Ibid., 153.

23. Ibid., 39–40.

24. Peter Leaney, Denes, e-mail message to author, September 8 & 9, 2004.

Chapter 15: Other Alternative Therapies

1. "How Does Acupuncture Work?" http://www.acupuncture.com (accessed November 11, 1999).

2. David J. Gilchrist, B.V.Sc., "An Introduction to Veterinary Acupuncture," AltVetMed Web site, http://www.altvetmed.org/pages/articles.html.

3. Susan Thorpe-Vargas and John C. Cargill, "Veterinary Acupuncture: Reaching the Point of Acceptance," *Acme Pet Newsletter,* http://www.acmepet.petsmart.com/ (site now discontinued).

4. David J. Gilchrist, B.V.Sc., "An Introduction to Veterinary Acupuncture," AltVetMed Web site, http://www.altvetmed.org/pages/articles.html.

5. Edward J. Boldt Jr., D.V.M., IVAS, e-mail message to author, November 1, 2004.

6. International Veterinary Acupuncture Society (IVAS) office, NA, e-mail message to author, August 24, 2004.

7. Are Thoresen, D.V.M., personal conversation, November 1999.

8. Ibid.

9. Are Thoresen, D.V.M., "Small Animal Cancer," Medical Acupuncture Web site, http://users.med.auth.gr/~karanik/english/webjour.htm.

10. Are Thoresen, D.V.M., personal conversation, November 1999.

11. Mary L. Brennan, D.V.M., with Norma Eckroate, *The Natural Dog: A Complete Guide for Caring Owners* (New York: Plume Books/Penguin, 1994), 157.

12. Andrew Weil, M.D., "Ask Dr. Weil," http://www.altmedicine.com (accessed November 18, 1999).

13. "Cancer Treatment: What Is the Role of Eastern Medicine?" *HealthFacts* 23 (July 1998): 4.

14. Tom Beckett and Marnie Reeder, "The Tellington Touch, The Touch That Heals," *Dog Owner's Guide* Web magazine, http://www.canismajor.com/ dog/ttouch.html (accessed December 10, 1999).

15. April Linville, D.V.M., and Susan Spalter, "More on TTouch: Tellington Touch Can Calm Nerves, Reduce Tension and Improve Quality of Life," *Dog Owner's Guide* Web magazine, http://www.canismajor.com/dog/ttouch2.html (accessed December 10, 1999).

16. Linda Tellington-Jones, "Tellington TTouch Equine Awareness Method and Tellington Ttouch Training," http://www.lindatellingtonjones.com.

17. Linville and Spalter, "More on TTouch," *Dog Owner's Guide* Web magazine, www.canismajor.com/dog/ttouch2.html.

18. Rita Reynolds, personal correspondence, February 2, 2000.

19. Ibid.

20. Reiki Home Page, "Welcome to Reiki," http://www.reiki.com.au.

21. Raphaela Pope, personal correspondence, April 21, 2000.

22. Ibid.

23. Jennah Dickinson, personal correspondence, April 20, 2000.

24. Jennah Dickinson, "Touch Your Dog," *DogStar* Web newsletter, February 6, 2000.

25. Maryann Struman, "Pet Healer Uses Ancient Japanese Method to Help Her Care for Animals," *Detroit News,* August 17, 1995.

26. University of Miami School of Medicine Department of Pediatrics, Touch Research Institute Web site, http://www.miami.edu/touch-research/.

27. TimeOut Corporate World Massage, "Touch Research Institute Synopsis," www.corpmassage.com.

Chapter 16: Pet Insurance and PPOs

1. "The Membership Savings Program for Pet Owners," Pet Assure (brochure), http://www.petassure.com.
2. U.S. Census Bureau, "Income, Poverty, and Health Insurance Coverage in the United States," http://www.census.gov/hhes/www/income.html (accessed December 13, 2004).
3. Jack Stephens, D.V.M., personal correspondence, January 3, 2000.
4. "Pet Insurance," *Petlife Magazine,* June 1999, 47.
5. "Americans Can Protect Best Friends from Cancer," Veterinary Pet Insurance press release, March 15, 1999.
6. Kathy Baumgardner, "Pet Health Insurance Continues to Gain Ground in Foreign Veterinary Markets," *DVM* Web news magazine, September 1997, http://www .dvmnewsmagazine.com.
7. "Insurance Avoidance," *Catnip,* May 1995, 3.
8. Mark Effenberg, e-mail message to author, September 16, 2004.
9. Healthy Pets Insurance Web site, http://www.healthy-pets.co.uk (accessed September 16, 2004).
10. Kathy Baumgardner, "Pet Health Insurance Continues to Gain Ground in Foreign Markets," *DVM* Web news magazine, September 1997, http://www.dvmnews magazine.com.
11. DBI Insurance Company literature, 1999.
12. Charles Nebenzahl, e-mail message to author, October 14, 2004.
13. Charles Nebenzahl, e-mail message to author, November 11, 2004.
14. Charles Nebenzahl, e-mail message to author, October 12, 2004.
15. Brakke Consulting, Inc., *Brakke Consulting* newsletter, December 17, 2004, http://www.brakkeconsulting.com.
16. Myrna Milani, D.V.M., e-mail message to author, February 10, 2005.

Chapter 17: If Your Pet Already Has Cancer

1. Richard H. Pitcairn, D.V.M., and Susan Hubble Pitcairn, *Dr. Pitcairn's Complete Guide to Natural Health for Dogs and Cats,* rev. ed. (Emmaus, Penn.: Rodale Press, 1995): 247.
2. "A Revolutionary Innovation in the Battle against Canine Cancer" (brochure), Hill's Pet Nutrition and personal conversation with Kelli Williams, Barkely Evergreen and Partners, September 29, 1999.
3. Norma Bennett Woolf, "Iams Nutrition Symposium Reveals Diet Connection to Major Illnesses: Implications for HumanDiet," *Dog Owner's Guide* Web magazine 1999 http://www.canismajor.com/dog.
4. Jason Vogel, "Top Dog," *Financial World* 164 (20 June 1995): 58.
5. Tara Parker-Pope, "Premium Pet Food: Is It Science or Marketing?" *Lexington Herald-Leader,* 1997.

6. Gregory K. Ogilvie, D.V.M., and Antony S. Moore, M.V.Sc., "Managing the Veterinary Cancer Patient: A Practice Manual," Veterinary Learning Systems, 28–30.

7. Mica DiAngelis, in discussion with the author, August 10, 2002.

8. Anita Frazier with Norma Eckroate, *The New Natural Cat: A Complete Guide for Finicky Owners,* rev. ed. (New York: Dutton/Penguin, 1990), 240.

9. Toni Eames and Ed Eames, "Partners in Independence," *DogWorld,* July 1993, 109.

10. Ed Eames, "Kirby, My Miracle Worker," *laJoie,* Winter 2000, 16–18.

11. Marilyn Putz, e-mail message to author, August 27, 2004.

Chapter 18: Pain Management for Animals

1. Companion Animal Pain Management Consortium, *The Essential Guide to Pain Management, A Complete Resource for Veterinary Pain Management,* 2004.

2. T. J. Dunn, D.V.M., "Managing Pain in Dogs," originally in *Dog World Magazine* February 2002, also available at http://www.thepetcenter.com/gen/pm.html (accessed August 19, 2004).

3. Rita Reynolds, e-mail message to author, August 18, 2004.

4. Reynolds, e-mail message to author, August 2004.

5. Amanda Katz and Patricia Collier, "Rainbow Trout Shown to Feel Pain," Wildlife News on Animal News Center, http://www.anc.org/wildlife/wildlife_article (accessed June 19, 2003).

6. Bev Mercer and Sue O'Brien, "Companion Animal Pain Management Consortium Created to Foster Education and Research in Animal Pain Management," Press Release for Pfizer Animal Health, December 21, 2000.

7. J. C. Brearley, VetMB, "Cancer Pain and Analgesia," from Proceedings of Association of Veterinary Soft Tissue Surgeons, Surgical Oncology, 17 and 18 October 2003, http://www.vet.cam.ac.uk/avsts/AVSTSProcOct2003pdf (accessed December 10, 2004).

8. Charles Short, D.V.M., "Companion Animal Pain Management Consortium Created to Foster Education and Research in Animal Pain Management," December 21, 2000.

9. French, VandeWoude, Granowski, and Maul, "An Example of Pain Assessment in Research Animals," *Assessment of Pain in Laboratory Animals,* Contemporary Topics 39:85, 2000, University of Florida—Animal Care & Use, http://iacuc .ufl.edu.

10. T. J. Dunn, D.V.M., "Managing Pain in Dogs."

11. Dr. J. C. Brearley, VetMB, "Cancer Pain and Analgesia," Proceedings of Surgical Oncology meeting held 17 and 18 October 2003 in Cambridge, U.K., http://www .vet.cam.ac.uk/avsts/AVSTSProcOct2003pdf (accessed December 10, 2004).

12. The Essential Tools for Pain Management—The Complete Veterinary Pain Management Kit, 2004.

13. J. Michael McFarland, D.V.M., e-mail message to author, September 15 and 16, 2004.

14.   Companion Animal Pain Management Consortium, "The Essential Guide to Pain Management, A Complete Resource for Veterinary Pain Management," 2004.

15.   Ibid.

16.   William Tranquilli, D.V.M., conversation with author, September 7, 2004.

17.   Ibid.

18.   Charles Short, D.V.M., *Management of Animal Pain, Course Syllabus,* Companion Animal Pain Management Consortium, Preface, 2002.

19.   Charles Short, D.V.M., e-mail message to author, October 2, 2004.

Chapter 19: Grieving and Accepting the Loss

1.   University of Pennsylvania's Cancer Center OncoLink Web site, http://www.oncolink.upenn.edu/specialty/vet_onc.

2.   Peter Gethers, *People Weekly* 51, May 31, 1999.

3.   "KSU Veterinary Clinic to Open Home-Like Consultation Room," Kansas State University News Services, April 29, 1999, http://www.newss.ksu.edu/

4.   Carolyn Ashton, personal correspondence, November 2, 1999.

5.   Donna Raditic, D.V.M., personal conversation, December 1999.

6.   Donna Raditic, e-mail message to author, November 8, 2004.

7.   Susan Hamlin, e-mail message to author, September 19, 2004.

8.   ASPCA Companion Animal Mourning Project Study, ASPCA Web site, http://www.aspca.org.

9.   George Page, *Inside the Animal Mind* (New York: Doubleday, 1999), 195.

10.   Kaetheryn Walker, *The Heart That Is Loved Never Forgets: Recovering from Loss: When Humans and Animals Lose Their Companions* (Rochester, Vt: Healing Arts Press, 1999), 75–79.

11.   Pet Grief Support Service, Companion Animal Association of Arizona, Inc., http://www.caaainc.org/petgriefsupport.htm.

12.   Carolyn Ashton, personal correspondence, November 2, 1999.

13.   Ibid.

14.   Andrea Spencer, National Cancer Society for Animals, e-mail messages to author, September 11 & October 4, 2004.

15.   Pet Education website, "National Pet Memorial Day: September 12, 2004," http://www.peteducation.com (accessed September 12, 2004).

16.   Lisa Rathke, "Times Argus offers obituaries for pets," *The Burlington Free Press,* August 2, 2004, section B.

17.   Gary Kowalski, *Goodbye, Friend: Healing Wisdom for Anyone Who Has Ever Lost a Pet* (Walpole, N.H.: Stillpoint Publishing, 1997), 17.

18.   Ibid., 15.

19.   Ibid., 13.

Index

BOOKS OF RELATED INTEREST

Homeopathic First Aid for Animals
Tales and Techniques from a Country Practitioner
by Kaetheryn Walker

The Heart That Is Loved Never Forgets
*Recovering from Loss: When Humans and
Animals Lose Their Companions*
by Kaetheryn Walker

How Animals Talk
And Other Pleasant Studies of Birds and Beasts
by William J. Long

Animal Voices
Telepathic Communication in the Web of Life
by Dawn Baumann Brunke

Awakening to Animal Voices
A Teen Guide to Telepathic Communication with All Life
by Dawn Baumann Brunke

Meditations with Animals
A Native American Bestiary
by Gerald Hausman

Dolphins and Their Power to Heal
by Amanda Cochrane and Karena Callen

Seven Experiments That Could Change the World
A Do-It-Yourself Guide to Revolutionary Science
by Rupert Sheldrake

Inner Traditions • Bear & Company
P.O. Box 388
Rochester, VT 05767
1-800-246-8648
www.InnerTraditions.com

Or contact your local bookseller